Hear **AND** Understand

Hear **AND** Understand

what you **NEED TO KNOW** about
HEARING LOSS and **HEARING AIDS**

ERIC FREDERICK, AuD

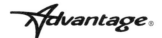

Published by Advantage, Charleston, South Carolina.
Member of Advantage Media Group.

ADVANTAGE is a registered trademark, and the Advantage colophon is a trademark of Advantage Media Group, Inc.

Printed in the United States of America.

ISBN: 978-1-59932-569-9
LCCN: 2016938618

This publication is designed to provide accurate and authoritative information in regard to the subject matter covered. It is sold with the understanding that the publisher is not engaged in rendering legal, accounting, or other professional services. If legal advice or other expert assistance is required, the services of a competent professional person should be sought.

Advantage Media Group is proud to be a part of the Tree Neutral® program. Tree Neutral offsets the number of trees consumed in the production and printing of this book by taking proactive steps such as planting trees in direct proportion to the number of trees used to print books. To learn more about Tree Neutral, please visit **www.treeneutral.com.** To learn more about Advantage's commitment to being a responsible steward of the environment, please visit **www.advantagefamily.com/green.**

Advantage Media Group is a publisher of business, self-improvement, and professional development books and online learning. We help entrepreneurs, business leaders, and professionals share their Stories, Passion, and Knowledge to help others Learn & Grow. Do you have a manuscript or book idea that you would like us to consider for publishing? Please visit **advantagefamily.com** or call **1.866.775.1696.**

To the thousands of patients who have entrusted me with improving their lives through better hearing. Your willingness to let me help you stay actively connected with your home, family, and community is a humbling inspiration every day.

TABLE OF CONTENTS

ABOUT THE AUTHOR

D r. Eric Frederick is an audiologist (AuD) with decades of work in nonprofit hearing clinics; hospitals; ear, nose, and throat surgery offices; and private-practice audiology. He has worked in research and in clinical practice. He earned his bachelor of arts degree in psychology from Indiana University in 1990; his master of science degree in audiology from Washington University in St. Louis in 1994; and his doctor of audiology degree from A.T. Still University of Health Sciences in 2002.

He has spent his time helping patients of all ages stay in touch with their world through better communication. He understands that hearing is not about just hearing speech but is about keeping each and every person in touch with the people who are most important around them. There's a well-known quote by Hellen Keller stating that if she had to choose which sense to lose, she would rather be blind then deaf because being blind cuts you off from a world of things, but being deaf cuts you off from a world of people.

Every day of his professional life, Dr. Frederick has followed his passion for restoring hearing to people to help them keep in touch with their important others. He is the founder and current owner of Audiology Center Northwest in Portland, Oregon. His clinic is open to the public, and if you would like to contact Dr. Frederick or his team, they are located at 919 Northeast 19th Avenue, Suite 170, Portland, OR, 97232. His phone number is 503-232-1845. His website is www.audiologycenternw.com, and e-mails may be directed to info@audiologycenternw.com.

FOREWORD

During my thirty-eight years of practice as an ear, nose, and throat specialist, I have seen many thousands of patients with hearing difficulties. Most patients' hearing loss falls into two broad categories: middle ear conditions, which can be treated medically or surgically, and inner ear conditions, which affect the vast majority of hearing-impaired patients.

The wider consequences of permanent hearing loss are poorly understood by the public, not fully appreciating the devastating effects such as producing feelings of isolation, despair, and depression, as well as being responsible for problems at work and affecting personal and family relationships.

Despite these deeply disturbing effects of hearing loss on both patients and their families, fewer than 20 percent of hearing-impaired people in the US are given the benefit of hearing aids, for a number of reasons. In some cases, they have been told, even by physicians (who should know better) that hearing aids will not help them or are too expensive or obtrusive. And because hearing loss is associated with aging, there is often resistance in accepting this truth.

In addition, there is now strong evidence, based on recent research, showing that patients with dementia of all degrees, with associated hearing loss, who tend to retreat into their own private worlds, can definitely benefit in their daily activities from hearing aids.

Delaying treatment for hearing loss can have permanent negative consequences on your health. By choosing to have your hearing loss accurately measured and effectively treated, your personal, work-related, and social life can be vastly improved. Surely you would like to feel more confident, more connected, and more independent—this book will tell you how!

There have been major advances in hearing aid design in recent years. This book will help you understand the conditions causing hearing loss, and for the millions who could truly benefit from hearing aids, the information in these pages will help you make wise decisions regarding your choice of hearing aid professional, help you interpret and understand your test results, and explain in detail the specific features of modern hearing aids, enabling you as a consumer to make educated decisions regarding your choice of hearing instruments.

If you have a hearing problem, or if any of your loved ones have been diagnosed with dementia and associated hearing loss, this book will help you understand every aspect of hearing impairment and the latest in effective treatment. You owe it to yourself to hear what you've been missing!

—Derek S. Lipman, MD

Ear, nose, and throat physician and author of

Snoring from A to ZZZZ: Proven Cures for the Night's Worst Nuisance

INTRODUCTION

I f you picked up this book, the chances are good that you or someone you care about is struggling to hear and understand speech. You are not alone. Hearing loss is one of the most common chronic health conditions in the United States, but it is an invisible disorder. When you have a hearing loss, it's not obvious—there's no wheelchair, no white cane. There's no external sign for people to know that you are struggling. In fact, even you may not know that you are struggling to hear and understand.

When you have a hearing loss, it progresses slowly most of the time. There's no pain to let you know that it's coming on. You just lose a little more clarity in your hearing every day until it builds up to a point where you finally have to admit that you have an issue—maybe it's not that everybody mumbles but that your hearing actually isn't quite what it used to be.

We used to say that hearing loss was the third most common chronic health condition, right after arthritis and high blood pressure. That was based on the assumption that 10 percent of the population had a significant hearing loss. We know now that the number is much, much higher. We had come to that 10 percent figure by simply asking people if they had a hearing loss. Doctors don't diagnose any other condition in health care by simply asking people if they have the condition. Your physician would never diagnose high blood pressure just by asking you if you had it. In addition, hearing loss comes on so slowly that many people don't know or suspect that they have a problem.

Johns Hopkins University recently did a study in which they randomly tested a large population to see who truly had hearing loss. The researchers found that close to 20 percent of the population over the age of twelve has a hearing loss in at least one ear.[1] By the time we're over the age of fifty, that number is upward of 25 percent. By the time we're eighty, we have approximately an 80 percent chance of having a hearing loss.

The problem is that our society has not caught up with this situation. Our medical community is not actively screening people for hearing loss or talking about how important it is. We know that hearing loss can have a devastating impact on quality of life and relationships. We know that it can have a massive impact on mental health, including depression and anxiety. And as you read this book you'll find that there is a link between hearing loss and dementia, Alzheimer's disease, memory loss, and cognitive decline.[2] Even though our medical system does not routinely test for hearing loss, you have taken an important first step by picking up this book. You've read this far, and I hope you will read more.

When you have a hearing loss, it starts out slowly. Most people don't even realize the loss because almost no one is completely deaf. Even those with a significant hearing loss can hear—they just can't understand. The reason is that hearing loss does not affect every pitch equally. It's common to have good hearing for low-pitched, bass sounds but very impaired hearing for high-frequency, high-pitched sounds.

When you have a high-pitched hearing loss, you'll hear but not understand. The reason is that those deep bass sounds that most

---

1 Frank R. Lin, John K. Niparko, Luigi Ferrucci, "Hearing loss prevalence in the United States," *Arch Intern Med*, 2011; 171 (20): 1851–1852.
2 Frank R. Lin, MD, PhD; E. Jeffrey Metter, MD; Richard J. O'Brien, MD, PhD; Susan M. Resnick, PhD; Alan B. Zonderman, PhD; Luigi Ferrucci, MD, PhD, "Hearing Loss and Incident Dementia," *Arch Neurol*, 2011; 68 (2): 214–220.

people can hear tend to be vowels, while the high-pitched, shrill, squeaky sounds that hearing loss takes away tend to be consonants. With most hearing losses, you can hear that someone is talking, but because you don't hear the high-pitched, brassy consonants like *s, f, t,* or *th*, you are constantly trying to put together a jigsaw puzzle with 30 percent of the pieces missing. That can be exhausting.

At the end of the day, you may feel ground down. You may frequently misunderstand speech. You may make funny mistakes, and people may laugh at you because you misheard something. These are the symptoms that we would expect with a high-frequency hearing loss. The good news is that this can almost always be improved through technology.

One of the things that drives me crazy as an audiologist is hearing a physician say to a patient, "You don't need help. You have a hearing loss, but it's normal for your age." Or, "You're eighty years old, so you *should* have a hearing loss." Or even, "You're sixty or seventy years old, so you should expect to have a hearing loss. It's normal."

This is one of the most limiting things that you as a patient can ever hear. Just because you have a hearing loss that is common to people of your age group does not mean that it should be ignored. No matter what your age, hearing loss can cut you off from the world. It puts you at risk for mental health disorders, it damages your relationships, and it reduces your earning potential in the work force.

If a disorder is a problem for people who are forty years old, it's also a problem for people who are seventy. Society does not give up on you just because you have started collecting your pension. There is no other medical disorder for which a doctor would tell you, "You're just old . . . deal with it." No physician would ever tell you, "You're eighty years old and have cataracts. Just stop reading, and deal with it." No, the doctor would step in and treat your cataracts to improve your vision. If a physician is telling you that hearing loss is normal for your age and that you should not do anything about it, it's time to see an expert in hearing loss instead of that physician.

Another thing that holds people back from getting hearing devices is the misperception that no one has success with them. Almost every day in my clinic I see new patients who know that they have a hearing loss and are not functioning well in their communication environment, yet they say something like: "I have a friend who has hearing aids, but they just sit in the drawer. Why would I want to get something that doesn't work?" Others say, "I bought a set of hearing aids over the Internet, and I feel like throwing them away. Why would another pair be any better?"

My answer to these patients is that properly fitted hearing aids actually have an extremely high satisfaction rate. The largest study done on hearing aid satisfaction, the MarkeTrak series of studies, shows that overall, hearing devices have an 85 percent satisfaction rate. That means that 85 percent of wearers are either satisfied or highly satisfied with their hearing devices. Technology continues to improve, and since the time that study was last done, we're finding that some devices can get as high as a 96 percent satisfaction rating.[3] That means that ninety-six out of every hundred people who try these devices rate themselves as satisfied.

Few products in the marketplace have this level of satisfaction—not cell phone service, not televisions, not cars, and not physical therapy. It's time for us to give up the myth that hearing devices don't work. Keep in mind, though, that not every single person is an appropriate candidate for hearing devices. Also remember that hearing aids need to be tailored to your individual hearing loss,

---

3 *Oticon Alta International Satisfaction Study,* Oticon, 2013, http://www.oticon.com/professionals/products-and-innovation/news/alta-satisfaction-study.aspx.

not purchased in a store or over the Internet. It is my hope that by reading this book, you'll learn the questions to ask when you visit a professional to find out if and how you might benefit—and change your life—with hearing aids.

For example, one of the most common questions is whether hearing aids can help hearing when there is background noise present. When you have a hearing loss, the most difficult listening environments are almost always moderately noisy areas such as restaurants, group meetings, family gatherings, or car travel. When people ask me whether hearing aids can help in these situations, I assure them that the answer is yes. Technology has come a long way from what you may remember. If you remember hearing aids that did not help with background noise, or if you had hearing aids in the past that weren't much help, it's time to come in and discuss this issue. Because hearing in noisy environments is such an important problem, we'll discuss it at length in chapter 7.

Another thing that keeps many people from investigating hearing devices is that they carry a cost—a cost in terms of both time and emotion but also a significant financial cost. Hearing aids are expensive. There's no other way to say it. But if you know your rights, which we will talk about throughout this book—particularly in chapter 8—you will come to understand how to minimize your financial risk.

One of the most important ways you can make sure you spend your money wisely is to understand that every hearing device dispensed in the United States comes with a money-back trial period. One of the primary purposes of this book is to help you, as a consumer, to understand what you can do to protect yourself and to get the most out of your hearing aid trial. You'll also learn about the warranty period, during which a hearing aid can be repaired at no cost, as well as loss and damage insurance that will cover you if your hearing aid becomes lost or catastrophically damaged. Getting a hearing device is an investment. Taking that step can be nerve-racking, but knowing your rights can put you back in control.

————

You may be reading this book now because you received it from your physician or your audiologist after a hearing test. You may have heard me speak on the subject of hearing loss and hearing devices.

You may have a feeling that your hearing is not what it once was. This is quite possible because a huge number of risk factors can set you up for a hearing loss. Our bodies are integrated systems. Our ears don't operate in isolation, and many health conditions that affect other parts of our bodies also affect our ears.

All of the following dramatically increase the likelihood that you will have a hearing loss: having cardiovascular disease, diabetes, or a family history of hearing loss; being a smoker; taking most medications that carry the risk of dizziness, hearing loss, or ringing in the ears; having erectile dysfunction and taking medication for it; or being exposed to either occupational or recreational noise, gunfire, or military service.

If you fit any of these descriptions—or if your doctor has told you that you might have a hearing loss—and you haven't had your hearing tested, it's time to pick up the phone and make a call. My hope for you is that in reading this book you will gain the knowledge to get back in the driver's seat. Until you know something about hearing loss and hearing aids, you will not even know where to begin or what questions to ask. By learning more—by educating yourself and reading this book—you will be able to be an integral part of the process when it is time for you to go in and get your hearing tested. You will know what questions are most important to ask as a patient, and you will be able to feel confident in asking them. Hearing aids can be a life-changing event. Getting hearing aids is a major life decision, and you need to be part of it.

It is likely that you have been thinking about your hearing for some time before choosing to pick up this book, wondering if your hearing loss is bad enough to address. One of the most surprising things you will read in this book may be the concept that you can actually be harmed by waiting too long to address your hearing loss. Back in the 1960s and 1970s, we used to say that you should wait as long as possible before getting hearing aids—that you should wait to seek help until your hearing is so bad that you cannot carry on a conversation anymore.

Current research suggests that this was terrible advice. There now appears to be a significant risk in waiting too long to correct hearing loss. In the United States, the average person waits seven years from the time they suspect a hearing loss to the time that they get their hearing tested. During that waiting period, what we're finding now is that the brain—the person's neurological system—is becoming less and less efficient at understanding the speech sounds that it's missing out on.

Your brain needs information to stay healthy, and information comes to it in the form of sensory input—in this case, sound. If you have a hearing loss, you are not feeding your brain the full diet of sounds it needs to stay healthy. Research has not yet determined whether hearing loss directly causes cognitive decline, dementia, or Alzheimer's disease, but we do see a strong link between hearing loss and some mental health disorders and quality-of-life issues.[4]

---

4 Sergei Kochkin and Carole M. Rogin, "Quantifying the Obvious: The Impact of Hearing Aids on Quality of Life," *Hearing Review*, 7 (January, 2000): 8–34.

I hope this book will encourage people to get their hearing tested sooner, so that they can make informed decisions about hearing devices. Hearing loss affects all aspects of life. Don't let it affect yours one day longer by putting off your hearing test!

———

I have spent more than twenty years helping people with hearing loss. I've worked with thousands of patients. Almost all of them have come in with some level of anxiety about the process, and I've found one thing to be true: most people want to know more. I've spent my adult life helping my patients learn more about why their hearing is affecting them the way it is, how technology can improve their hearing problem, and what the limits of technology might be.

A book can never be a substitute for face-to-face conversation with your clinical audiologist, but I hope this will be a starting point for you. It is my opportunity to tell you what I think are the most important issues that you need to know to put you back in control.

We begin in chapter 1, where I answer the question, "How am I harmed by waiting too long for hearing aids?" Once you've learned the benefits of hearing aids, chapter 2 answers what is probably your most important question: "How can I choose a great audiologist?"

Once you've chosen a provider, you might be wondering what to expect at your first visits to the audiologist. Chapter 3 explains what will happen when you visit your provider. You'll most likely have a hearing test during that visit, and chapter 4 will take you through that process step by step and tell you how to interpret the results.

The correction of hearing loss is complicated. Many people expect it to parallel the process of getting glasses and are surprised at the differences. Chapter 5 discusses why hearing loss is harder to correct than vision problems.

Chapter 6 covers the types of help that are available for hearing loss, and chapter 7 explains how hearing aids work.

As I've noted, hearing aids are expensive. Chapter 8 helps you be in control and minimize your risks by discussing the costs and legal protections you have when you purchase hearing aids. By the time you've absorbed all this information, you may be wondering, *Will hearing aids really help me?* The chapter also reassures you that contacting an audiologist may be the best move you can make.

Treating hearing loss is an extremely individual process. You are a unique person, and to get the most out of your hearing treatment, you need to talk with a professional who can uncover your particular needs as you communicate in the world.

Take ownership of your hearing loss. You've taken the first step by taking the initiative to pick this book up and start reading. That means that you are in the small minority of people who are taking action to help themselves hear better.

I am honored that you took the time to begin reading this book. I know that you'll have a lot of other questions as you read, but I've tried to anticipate as many of them as I can so that I can answer them along the way.

If you have any questions or wish to discuss anything in this book in more detail and are in the Portland, Oregon, area please call my office. We would be happy to see you and consult with you about your particular needs. And if you are in another part of the country, I cannot encourage you strongly enough to visit an audiologist's office locally and discuss your hearing problems and needs. Remember, you are in control of your health care.

CHAPTER 1

How Am I Harmed by Waiting Too Long for Hearing Aids?

Untreated hearing loss can have wide-ranging, serious effects on your life—effects that you may not even have thought of.

There are some major high-tech industries in my area, and one of my patients—who I'll call Stephen—works for a prominent microchip manufacturer. Stephen told me that he wasn't able to function in work meetings, because he wasn't able to hear in noisy environments where multiple people were talking.

He was becoming concerned because he had become stagnant in his position. Even though he had a high level of skill, he had been passed over for new promotions. He had lost some clients and messed up a few projects because, he felt, of his inability to hear. Stephen's income had suffered, and now his marriage was strained, due both to the loss of his income and to communication difficulties with his wife.

We talked through his needs and made sure his wife, Jan, was in on the process. Jan was enthusiastic about getting him the help that he needed. Once we put hearing devices on him, his entire life changed. He was much more confident at work. He was able to function well in work meetings, on the phone, and in face-to-face conversations.

Stephen's been promoted. Jan says their marriage has been great because now he can hear her in restaurants. They can go out and do the things they used to enjoy doing together—things that bonded them. Jan feels valued because Stephen stepped up and took the action and responsibility to do what he could for his hearing. And they're doing things that they never thought would be important to them before—such as traveling to Europe, which they'd avoided because he wouldn't have been able to hear the tour guide and thus wouldn't have enjoyed the trip.

Hearing loss touches every aspect of our lives in ways that we cannot even imagine until we correct it. Although I'm not a licensed psychologist, social worker, or counselor, I can say that I have had a huge number of people come in and tell me that I saved or improved their marriages.

You probably picked up this book because you're wondering if hearing aids can help you. You may feel you have a hearing loss, or your doctor may have recommended that you look into hearing aids.

Before you read on, you may want to begin by taking the following quiz to see if you might benefit from hearing aids.

Do you feel that you have difficulties hearing, or are you curious about possible symptoms of hearing loss? Then take this short evaluation. It's quick, painless, and easy, and it could be your first step to better hearing and living life to its fullest. (This checklist does not replace a professional hearing test, but the results might indicate whether or not it is worth seeking advice from an audiologist.)

1. Do people seem to mumble or speak in a softer voice than they used to?

2. Do you feel tired or irritable after a long conversation?

3. Do you sometimes miss key words in a sentence or frequently need to ask people to repeat themselves?

4. When you are in a group or in a crowded restaurant, is it difficult for you to follow the conversation?

5. When you are together with other people, does background noise bother you?

6. Do you often need to turn up the volume on your TV or radio?

7. Do you find it difficult to hear the doorbell or the telephone ring?

8. Is it difficult to carry on a telephone conversation?

9. Do you find it challenging to pinpoint the location of an object, such as an alarm clock or telephone, from the noise it makes?

10. Has someone close to you mentioned that you might have a problem with your hearing?

If you have answered yes to two or more of the above questions, you will benefit from a hearing consultation. Don't delay. If left untreated, hearing loss is associated with loss of income, relationship difficulties, depression, fatigue, possible dementia, and much more. You are too young to be struggling with all that. Want to hear more? Call your audiologist today for a hearing check-up.

Why should I get hearing aids now instead of waiting a couple of years?

This book's aim is to provide "answers to all your questions." I suspect, though, that "How am I harmed by waiting too long for hearing aids" isn't one of those questions. Please read on. This topic is important to the success of your hearing aids.

It's almost always easier to get adjusted to hearing aids sooner rather than later. The main reason is that you hear with your brain, not your ears. You don't actually hear a sound until the signal gets sent from your ear up to your brain.

Unfortunately, the cells in your brain require a steady diet of stimulation in order to stay healthy. If you go for years without stimulating the brain cells (called neurons) that receive signals from your ears, these cells will actually degrade and atrophy, or waste away, over time. Your brain is almost like a muscle. If you don't use it and exercise it, it gets weaker over time. The connections between the neurons in your brain can become weaker. Cells in your brain can actually die off or get reassigned from one task, such as hearing, to another task.

We often see patients who have put off the process of getting hearing aids for years or decades. Most people, in fact, wait about seven years before seeking help for a hearing loss. They have essentially been starving their brains of input.

If you do not address a hearing loss over time, it's not that the hearing loss will get more severe. You don't necessarily lose your ability to hear soft sounds by delaying treatment with hearing aids. What happens is that your ability to understand speech frequently becomes worse. Your ability to hear in difficult listening conditions—amid background noise, for example—also often becomes worse.

One way we've found out about the changes that occur over time is by studying people who have a hearing loss in both ears but who get a hearing aid in just one ear—usually for financial reasons. Their understanding of speech in the unaided ear tends to degrade faster than in the aided ear.[5] Their ability to understand speech tends to get worse in the ear that is not used as much. We think that this is because the brain's ability to process signals from that ear gets worse over time. The brain cells that are responsible for understanding speech on the unaided side aren't being used and eventually weaken or even die off.

We do find that if we put a hearing aid on the unaided ear at a later date, the person will recover some neurologic function. The hearing aid, though, is never quite as efficient as it would have been

---

5 S. Silman, S.A. Gelfand, C.A. Silverman, "Late-onset auditory deprivation: effects of monaural versus binaural hearing aids," *Journal of the Acoustical Society of America*, Nov. 1984; 76 (5): 1357–62.

if the hearing device had been in that ear earlier. It also takes much longer for the person to regain the function in the ear that went a long time without a hearing aid.

It logically follows that when someone with a hearing loss doesn't have a hearing aid in either ear, this same type of nerve cell degeneration occurs for both ears. The problem is that it takes a long time to get the neurologic function back, and it may never come back fully. The rule of thumb is that for every year you go without hearing aids, it will take you approximately a month to get back to your best neurologic function.

I've heard that hearing loss may be related to dementia. Is there any truth to that?

A growing body of research from John Hopkins University demonstrates a definite relationship between hearing loss and cognitive decline such as dementia, memory loss, and Alzheimer's disease.[6] It appears that approximately 30 percent of age-related cognitive decline is related to hearing loss. Please note that I've said there's a *relationship* between hearing loss and some kinds of cognitive decline. We do not have enough data to say that hearing loss causes dementia or other kinds of cognitive decline, but there certainly is a relationship.

The hearing loss tends to occur first, and the cognitive loss follows. If you have a mild hearing loss that is untreated, you are at twice the risk of having dementia or other cognitive decline. If you have, say, a moderate hearing loss that's untreated, you have three times the risk of dementia. And if you have a severe hearing loss that's untreated, you have five times the risk of dementia.

---

6 Lin, "Hearing Loss and Incident Dementia," 214–220.

Another way to say this is that on average, every 10 decibels (abbreviated dB) of hearing loss you experience gives you a 20 percent increase in the possibility of having dementia or cognitive decline. Every 25 dB of untreated hearing loss adds seven years to your cognitive age. So if you have a 50 dB hearing loss that you haven't treated and you're an eighty-year-old, you're creating a brain age of ninety-four. This is a big deal! None of us wants to experience dementia, memory loss, or other cognitive issues any sooner than we have to.

I wish we could say with certainty that hearing aids will help delay cognitive decline, but we don't have the research to definitively say that yet. Studies are being done as this is being written to determine whether treating a hearing loss with hearing aids can help delay the onset of dementia or memory loss. The most important research on this topic is a long-term, twenty-five-year study.[7] In this study, groups of people who thought their hearing was normal were compared with one group who thought they had a hearing loss but *did* wear hearing aids and another group who thought they had hearing loss but *did not* wear hearing aids.

These three groups were compared over twenty-five years of their lives. The authors reported that the groups who reported either normal hearing or who reported using hearing aids to treat their hearing loss had the same level of mental/cognitive ability throughout the twenty-five-year period. By comparison, *the group that reported that they had a hearing loss but did not wear hearing aids lost more mental/cognitive ability over time.*

Science and statistics can be hard to interpret sometimes. We cannot always say that one thing causes the other. What we do know

---

7 H. Amieva, C. Ouvrard, C. Giulioli, C. Meillon, L. Rullier, J. F. Dartigues, "Self-Reported Hearing Loss, Hearing Aids, and Cognitive Decline in Elderly Adults: A 25-Year Study," *Journal of the American Geriatrics Society*, 63 (October 2015): 2099–2104.

at this point is that hearing loss is a definite predictor of cognitive decline. We also know that hearing aids may possibly have the potential to help put off cognitive decline—although it's important to keep in mind that this has not yet been scientifically proven.

How can hearing aids make my life richer?

In 1999, the National Council on Aging did a wonderful study on the effects of untreated hearing loss. They gathered over 2,300 hearing-impaired people and split them into two groups. In one group were people who had a hearing loss and opted to treat their hearing loss with hearing aids. In the other group were people who had hearing loss but opted not to treat their hearing loss with hearing aids.

The researchers then asked both groups of people—the hearing aid users and nonusers—questions about more than a hundred quality-of-life indicators. They asked them about their social relationships, work function, depression, anxiety, paranoia, self-esteem, overall satisfaction with life, social isolation, irritability, and fatigue. They found that on almost every one of these indicators, the group of people who opted to treat their hearing loss with hearing aids did better than the group who opted not to treat their hearing loss.

This really points up the fact that hearing aids aren't just about making sounds louder. They aren't even just about making you better able to understand speech. Hearing aids are about making your life better—helping you to be the person you see yourself as, the person you want to be.

The people in the study felt that, because of their hearing aids, their relationships were better. They felt that their hearing aids gave them higher self-esteem or higher quality of life.

If you can communicate better, you're more likely to be more social. You're more likely to feel more confident. You're more likely to perform better at work. If you perform better at work, you're more likely to make more money. You're more likely to be active in your community or engaged with your family. Hearing aids are about changing how you walk through the world.

A small percentage of people in the study even said that their love life got better after getting hearing aids. This little fact really shows just how far-reaching the ability to hear can be in our lives. After all, hearing aids are about connecting with other people, letting you get in touch with people. And if you can connect and communicate and stay in touch with your family more, you're more likely to be a better partner to your spouse. It's not surprising that your romantic relationships will get better if you're more responsive to your partner. After all, the best things we say to each other in life are said in a whisper, not in a shout.

How can I be more in charge of my hearing health?

It's your job, as the director of your own health care, to understand that many health conditions can cause hearing loss. In fact, your physician may not know about some of them. It's up to you to take a proactive stand and bring this topic up with your doctor.

RISK FACTORS FOR HEARING LOSS

You may be at greater risk for hearing loss if any of the following apply to you:

- have diabetes
- have cardiovascular disease
- have kidney disease
- take certain medications, such as Viagra
- have a history of smoking
- have a history of alcohol abuse

Hearing loss may put you at risk for the following:

- decreased cognitive function
- depression
- falling
- decreased earnings at work

Diabetes doubles your chance of hearing loss.[8] Prediabetes also doubles your chance of hearing loss, as does kidney disease.[9] Many cardiovascular diseases, or heart disease, triple your chance of

---

8 "Diabetes and Hearing Loss," American Diabetes Association, 2016, http://www.diabetes.org/living-with-diabetes/treatment-and-care/seniors/diabetes-and-hearing-loss.html.

9 "Hearing Loss Linked to Moderate Chronic Kidney Disease," National Kidney Foundation, 2016, https://www.kidney.org/news/ekidney/november10/HearingLoss_November10.

hearing loss.[10] Smoking also increases your chance of hearing loss, and hearing loss frequently even causes depression.[11]

Alcohol is linked with hearing loss, as are many medications. For example, Viagra doubles your chance of hearing loss,[12] and two doses a week of Tylenol or other over-the-counter pain relievers can also double your chance of hearing loss.[13]

If you have chronic pain, kidney disease, heart disease, diabetes, or any of these other risk factors, it's up to you to go to your doctor and say that you want regular hearing testing. There's no reason for hearing loss to rob you of years of connection with the people who are most important to you.

Your physician may not realize all of these links between health conditions and hearing loss. Primary-care doctors have a lot on their plate and don't always have hearing loss on their radar screen. You need to feel empowered; go in and tell your physician that you've read this book and understand that there's a link between some health conditions and hearing loss. Ask that your doctor refer you for hearing testing on a regular basis. Take charge of your hearing health!

---

10 R. H. Hull, S. R. Kerschen, "The Influence of Cardiovascular Health on Peripheral and Central Auditory Function in Adults: A Research Review," *American Journal of Audiology*, 19 (June 2010) 9–16.

11 Karen J. Cruickshanks, PhD; Ronald Klein, MD; Barbara E. K. Klein, MD; Terry L. Wiley, PhD; David M. Nondahl, MS; Ted S. Tweed, MS, "Cigarette Smoking and Hearing Loss: The Epidemiology of Hearing Loss Study," *JAMA*. 1998; 279 (21): 1715–1719.

12 McGwin Jr, MS, PhD, "Phosphodiesterase Type 5 Inhibitor Use and Hearing Impairment," *Archives of Otolaryngology—Head and Neck Surgery*, 2010; 136 (5): 488.

13 Sharon G. Curhan, MD, ScM; Roland Eavey, MD; Josef Shargorodsky, MD; Gary C. Curhan, MD, ScD, "Analgesic Use and the Risk of Hearing Loss in Men," *American Journal of Medicine*, Mar. 2010; 123(3): 231–237.

CHAPTER 2

How Can I Choose a Great Audiologist?

In choosing a hearing aid, probably the most important thing that you can do as a patient is to choose the right person to get your hearing aid from.

One of my patients, who I'll call Tammy, was a perfect case in point. I met her when I was doing some public speaking; she came up to me and told me about her last experience. She was in her early fifties and had purchased hearing aids about a year before. But she had never been happy with them. She'd been back to her provider several times to try to make the hearing aids right, but she always felt that she heard better without them, and she was never really at ease with her provider.

Tammy came to me at the end of the talk and asked, "Eric, you seem like you know what you're doing. Would you be willing to take a look at my hearing aids and see if they can be made better for me?"

I said, "I'd be happy to do it. I'll start with a hearing test, and then we'll figure out what to do from there." The first time I saw her for the hearing test, I found out why she was unhappy. It turned out her hearing was normal.

She had been convinced by a hearing aid dealer to spend thousands of dollars on devices she didn't need. This, unfortunately, is one of the horror stories that we occasionally hear, and it's one of the reasons why hearing aids get such a bad reputation. There are different types of professionals who fit hearing aids, and Tammy went to somebody who was not a medical professional. The hearing aid dealer she saw was a commissioned salesperson, whose income depended solely on how much money customers spent.

The hearing aid dealer talked her into buying something she didn't need and then kept convincing her that if she just came in for one more adjustment, everything would be perfect, until she was beyond the point where she could return the hearing aids for a refund. By the time I saw her, she intuitively knew what the situation was. She knew that if she was hearing better without the hearing aids than with them, she never needed them in the first place.

In the end, I had to deliver the bad news that there was no way to make the hearing aids better for her. Instead, she needed to hold onto them until she actually had a hearing loss, and then we could make the hearing aids work for her. She was disappointed that she had spent the money but was relieved that she didn't have the same experience with me—that I didn't tell her everything would be okay if she just spent some more money. In retrospect, Tammy realized that she had never been comfortable with the first provider. She'd always felt pressured to purchase something rather than to understand her hearing loss. If she had understood how to interpret her test results, which we'll discuss in chapter 4, she never would have been in that position.

Choosing a professional to get your advice from is probably the most important single choice you have in getting treatment for your hearing loss. In the following pages, we will explore how to stack the deck in your favor when deciding who should advise you.

I think I may have a hearing loss. What should I do first?

If you suspect you have a hearing loss, you may be feeling overwhelmed with the number of choices. You may know various people with different kinds of hearing aids, and you may have noticed that there are different types of providers. What are the differences among them, and how do you choose? This chapter will give you the information and guidance you'll need.

It's important to keep in mind that when you buy hearing aids, you are a consumer, and you can be an active part of the process. By reading this book, you will find out how to be an informed consumer and learn what kinds of questions to ask that will lead you to a successful outcome.

What kinds of specialists treat people with hearing loss?

When you start the process of selecting a provider, it's often hard to know exactly what type of professional to see. There are really different types of professionals who deal with hearing loss: an ear, nose, and throat physician; an audiologist; and a hearing instrument specialist (or hearing aid dealer).

When should I visit an ear, nose, and throat physician?

The most visible and well known of the professionals who treat people with hearing loss are ear, nose, and throat physicians or ENTs—also sometimes called otolaryngologists. If they specialize just in ears, they are called otologists. If they specialize in the ear and the brain, they are called neurotologists. All of these professionals are medical doctors. They've been to medical school and have been trained in treating hearing loss with medications and surgery. If you have a type of hearing loss that will respond well to medication or surgery, an ear, nose, and throat physician should absolutely be involved and should be the team leader in your treatment.

You should see an ENT as soon as possible if your hearing loss came on suddenly; for example, if you woke up one day and your hearing was much worse than the day before. This kind of hearing loss may respond very well to medication but only if it's given in the early stages.

If there's a large difference between the hearing in your two ears, an ENT physician should be involved to determine why. The physician may use an imaging study of the head or neck, such as an MRI or a CT scan, to decide whether an anatomical difference explains the asymmetry of hearing.

In addition, if you're having pain in the ear, liquid draining from your ear, bleeding from your ear, significant dizziness, or a feeling of pressure in the ear, an ENT should be immediately involved in your care.

When should I visit an audiologist?

The reality, however, is that according to the Better Hearing Institute in Washington, DC, only about 10 percent of hearing losses at any given time respond well to medication or surgery.[14] The other 90 percent are permanent. The vast majority of people have a long-standing, gradually progressing hearing loss, and these people are best served by seeing an audiologist first.

Audiologists are highly trained professionals who have had anywhere from six to eight years of college to earn the title of audiologist. All audiologists coming into the field today need a doctorate degree. They typically have an AuD degree, which stands for doctor of audiology. You may find an older audiologist with a PhD or a master's degree.

Audiologists usually receive four years of training through a university following four years of undergraduate work in speech and hearing sciences. Their training encompasses hearing loss, anatomy and physiology, rehabilitation techniques, and hearing devices. In addition, audiologists are trained to help identify many medical conditions that are better treated by an ear, nose, and throat physician. If you start by consulting an audiologist to assess possible hearing loss, he or she has the training to guide you to an ENT in the event you would be better served by such a specialist. You can feel confident that audiologists have a strong basis of education to do their job.

It's also fine if you decide to begin by going to an ENT. Almost every ear, nose, and throat physician either has an audiologist on staff or he or she can refer patients to one. To treat hearing loss, ENTs need to be able to diagnose it. They do so through a hearing test, which is typically performed by an audiologist.

---

14 "Myths about Hearing Loss," Better Hearing Institute, http://www.betterhearing.org/hearingpedia/myths-about-hearing-loss.

As an audiologist, I never discourage patients from getting a medical second opinion from an ENT. The two professions work very well hand in hand. ENTs cover the medical side, and audiologists cover the rehabilitation side, so each professional knows something that the other one does not. As a starting point, though, most people will be served very well by beginning with a hearing test and then being referred to a primary care physician or an ear, nose, and throat physician if the audiologist finds that medical treatment might be helpful.

Should I ever choose to visit a hearing aid specialist or hearing aid dealer?

The third category of professionals who work with hearing loss and hearing aids are called hearing instrument specialists, hearing aid dispensers, hearing aid dealers, or even audioprosthetologists. In essence, they are all the same thing. The state you live in will determine this professional's title.

This category of professional is much more loosely regulated than ear, nose, and throat physicians and audiologists. Hearing instrument specialists are generally governed by state law, and states vary greatly in the amount of training that they require. For example, I practice in Oregon, only about ten minutes away from the state of Washington. An Oregon-based hearing instrument specialist by law must have two years more training than a Washington-based one, just one state over.

There are many very good hearing instrument specialists. However, keep in mind that these providers will have a much more variable course of training than you'll find with either an audiologist or an ear, nose, and throat physician. Most of the excellent hearing instrument specialists that I have encountered are fantastic at their jobs because they've gone above and beyond what the state requires for training.

How do I choose between an audiologist and a hearing instrument specialist to help with my hearing loss?

If you live in an area with access to both audiologists and hearing instrument specialists, why not stack the cards in your favor by going to somebody with more extensive education? An audiologist will virtually always have a much higher level of education than a hearing aid dealer.

If you do not live in an area with access to audiologists, be sure to find the most qualified hearing instrument specialist you can. One way to do so is to look for the letters *BC-HIS* after the person's name. *BC* stands for board certified, and *HIS* stands for hearing instrument specialist. These providers have voluntarily gotten additional training and undergone a nationwide certification program for hearing instrument specialists.

In some states, including my state of Oregon, ear, nose, and throat physicians and audiologists are categorized as medical professionals, while hearing instrument specialists are categorized as retail salespeople. Because of the differences in training and business models, you may have a very different experience with an ENT or audiologist than with a hearing instrument specialist.

If you're the type of person who thrives in the health-care system, you might choose to begin with an ENT or an audiologist. This might suit you if you see hearing loss as a medical condition that needs to be treated as such.

If instead you thrive in a retail model, you may prefer to feel like a customer rather than a patient. You may want to go where you can negotiate the price of a hearing aid, which audiologists cannot do—in fact, no provider who bills insurance companies can negotiate prices. If a provider who accepts insurance coverage lowers his cost on a device through haggling, this is considered insurance fraud with possible fines and jail time as a punishment. You as the patient should be extremely wary if your hearing aid provider starts offering discounts when you express reluctance to make a purchase decision.

Should I buy hearing aids over the Internet?

Recently, more and more companies sell hearing aids over the Internet. This means they sell to prospective patients they've never seen and recommend hearing devices for patients they've never tested. Some do have the patient send in a hearing test performed by an audiologist; someone looks at those test results and recommends a device that might be reasonably appropriate.

The problem here is that buying a hearing aid is not like buying a toaster or other appliance. Getting a hearing device is much more than just getting a product. The product itself—the hearing aid—accounts for only a small part of your success in using it. A hearing device is basically a blank slate. It must be programmed by a professional, who tells it how to behave when sound is coming in. The programming allows the hearing device to process sound and shape that sound in such a way that it gives you optimum speech understanding while keeping things as comfortable as possible. This programming is as unique to you as your eyeglass prescription and will not sound right to someone else.

Ideally, we want soft speech to be audible, moderate speech to be comfortable and loud speech to be tolerable. At the same time, we want to make speech as clear as possible while keeping background noise to a minimum. This is a very complicated process; it's not something that you can do well right out of the box. The process of getting a hearing device is very much like physical therapy. Your ability to process sound will change over time as you use the hearing device. It's like building muscle. You'll be able to distinguish sounds after a month of hearing aid wear that you could not have recognized on the first day.

There is a dance that happens between the hearing device and the patient. As the patient gets more capable, the device should deliver more to meet that capability. As part of the hearing aid fitting process, you are going to need to go back to the dispensing professional a few times. Three to four times is pretty typical in the first couple of months because your brain itself will change as it gets more experience with sounds that it hasn't experienced in years. You'll become a more efficient listener over time. And you'll want to feed your more-efficient brain a higher-quality signal so that you understand still more speech.

You can't get these adjustments if you purchase hearing aids over the Internet. You need to work with a professional you can visit for adjustments.

I see much lower prices for hearing aids in magazines and newspapers. Should I look into them?

It may be tempting to try to choose a hearing aid provider based on advertisements you see in newspapers or magazines. Beware: Buying hearing aids because their provider offers a low price can be one of the riskiest ways to pick a health-care provider.

Businesses pay many thousands of dollars to run flashy ads. Who pays for these ads? It's you, the patient, who pays. When you buy hearing aids from providers who buy these ads, you are paying their advertising budget.

In addition, the highest-quality, best-educated providers don't have to advertise aggressively in most communities. They get more than enough business through physician referrals and word of mouth from satisfied customers. These providers have treated patients well, so their patients recommend them to their friends. If a provider has to rely on large, flashy advertisements, you have to ask yourself why the business is not already full.

You may see what seem like amazing prices in advertisements. You may see two-for-one specials or $1,000-off deals. Think about it, though: if the hearing aids are a thousand dollars off or are half-priced in a two-for-one special, the business may well have to overcharge people regularly to be able to bring the prices down that much.

If you call around and ask about prices, be very wary of any place that has much higher or much lower prices than everyone else. If you call five places and one of them is twice as expensive as everyone else, cross that provider off the list. Similarly, if you call five different places and one quotes you prices that are half of what everyone else charges, you need to be wary. Providers that quote or advertise extremely low prices probably have some hidden costs. When you go in, you may find that a lot of things are not included in the price you were quoted. For example, the impression of your ear to fit your hearing aids might not be included. Or the price might include only one or two visits, when actually you'll need several more. Or your warranty may be very short. Or you may not have as long a time to return the hearing aids for a refund. Or, if you do return them for a refund, there may be extremely high restocking fees for which you will be responsible.

In my local area here in Portland, the price for the same hearing device from all the reputable sources does not vary more than 5 or 10 percent. The reason is that most reputable providers charge what it actually costs to dispense a hearing device. They don't pad the bill, and they are very up front about costs.

In the hearing aid world, as in the world in general, you'll tend to get what you pay for. And you'll find that the most reputable people are all charging what it really costs to get you the hearing aids that work best for you.

Some of my friends are not happy with their hearing aids. Is anyone really going to be able to fix my hearing anyway?

As an audiologist, I hear this over and over: "My friends say their hearing aids don't help much. Are hearing aids really something I want to pursue?"

The average patient coming in for a hearing test has waited seven years before getting tested. Most patients have known they have problems with hearing but have put off doing anything about it until they just can't stand it anymore. They may feel they are less happy with their social life or their professional life because of their hearing loss.

Many people look for excuses not to do something about their hearing problems. One of the biggest excuses they find is that they know people who have had bad experiences with hearing aids. They may have friends who keep their hearing aids in a drawer because they do not like them or know people who complain about not hearing well with their devices.

But remember that most people who talk about their experiences are people who are unhappy with them. Think back over the last month. How often did you tell somebody how wonderful it was that your feet, ankles, and legs work? That you could walk across the room without any pain—that it was a miracle of biology that you could get from here to there on your feet? We never tell anybody about our body's successes. But if we sprain an ankle, we tell everyone who listens how much pain we feel.

The same thing happens with hearing aids. The people who are happy with their experiences are generally the silent majority. The people who are unhappy, or who haven't been dealt with fairly by their providers, will tell everyone. And honestly, they *should* tell people. That's one of the ways people like you can figure out whether a prospective provider is a good or a bad risk. If you know five people who have had a negative experience with the same business, you'll know not to go there.

Some people have horror stories because they encountered a bad provider or malpractice or because their hearing loss is not the kind that can be helped with hearing aids. Some kinds of hearing loss are not correctable with hearing devices. However, a good provider should be able to identify whether a person is a good candidate for hearing aids and will not dispense them if they will not help the person hear better. On the whole, the vast majority of people are happy with their hearing aid provider. The horror stories we have spoken about really are the exception, not the rule.

Remember, if your friends are not satisfied with their hearing aids, don't think, *There's no point in getting hearing aids.* Instead think, *I won't get my hearing assessed by that provider.*

Hearing aids on the whole have an extremely high success rate. Approximately 81 percent of people who own hearing aids report being either satisfied or very satisfied.[15] This rate compares favorably with almost any other consumer product. In fact, hearing aids have a higher satisfaction rate than cars, TVs, cell phone service, gourmet coffees, physical therapy, and Internet providers and almost as high a satisfaction rate as Lasik surgery for the eyes, which is considered to be a near-perfect medical treatment.

In fact, certain hearing devices have up to a 96 percent satisfaction rate. That is absolutely phenomenal. There is almost nothing in this world that produces a 96 percent satisfaction rate. And there is certainly nothing else I know of that creates a 96 percent satisfaction rate but still has the widespread public perception that it doesn't work. If you have hearing loss, you owe it to yourself not to believe what everyone tells you but to go in and listen for yourself.

How can I choose the right provider and not get ripped off?

In the end, you need to pick a provider and a hearing device that works for you, and the only person who can determine that is you.

You'd do well to begin by asking other people what their experience has been with their providers. Ask your friends whom they use, and ask your physicians whom they would recommend.

When you begin to select among recommended providers, the most important thing to ask them is, "What options will I have to experience the device first?" You should be able to try a hearing device in the office before you even decide whether to order one. After all, you test-drive a car before you buy it; why shouldn't you be able to test-drive your hearing aids? In addition, the provider should give you a period of time when you can try the hearing device and return

---

15 H. B. Abrams, J. Kihm, "An Introduction to MarkeTrak IX: A New Baseline for the Hearing Aid Market," *Hearing Review*, 2015; 22(6): 16.

it for a refund. A competent provider will give you different ways that you, as the patient sitting in the chair, can understand and experience what you're getting into before you spend your money.

When I advise people how to pick a provider, I give some rules of thumb that are almost exactly what AARP recommends.[16]

1. *If possible, go to an audiologist for your hearing tests.* Audiologists have the highest level of training in hearing loss and how to treat it with devices.

2. *Make sure that you get your hearing tested in a sound-treated booth or room.* The office must have a dedicated space to run the hearing test in a very quiet environment. There must be a sound enclosure to isolate you and test your hearing in a quiet environment, not in a noisy office.

3. *Go to an audiologist who works with multiple brands of hearing aids instead of just one or two.* Some hearing aid providers have a financial arrangement with a certain manufacturer—they are either owned or funded by the manufacturer, and they can only order one brand of product. That's not always the best thing for a patient. Each manufacturer has its own philosophy

16 Consumer Guide to Hearing Aids, AARP, 2007.

and strategy for how to deal with hearing loss. Being able to select from a wide variety of products means that a provider can handle a wide variety of patients with many kinds of hearing losses. The provider should choose what's right for you, not force you to take what a particular manufacturer produces. You are an individual, and your provider should treat you as such.

4. *The audiologist should make sure that you are getting the most benefit from your hearing devices.* At the least, they should ensure that you are actually performing better with the hearing aids on than with them off. Too many providers simply take what the manufacturer recommends for your hearing loss, put the devices on your ears, and tell you to get used to them. This is generally what one would experience with Internet sales as well. That should never happen. When you are getting hearing health care, you are the most important person in the room. Your provider should sit down with you and make sure that the sound that is being delivered to you is making you communicate more effectively and keeping you comfortable.

5. *The audiologist should always take enough time with you.* He or she should talk with you in depth about how to use the hearing aids, how to adapt to them, and how to maintain them. Although it's not a terribly difficult process, learning to use and maintain hearing aids does take some practice. It doesn't feel natural on day one. You will no doubt have some questions during the first month or two. If you ever get the idea that your provider doesn't have time for you after you've written the check, that might not be the right person to continue working with.

Every hearing aid sold in the United States has at least a thirty-day trial period. If you're not happy with your provider during your trial period, return the hearing aids and find a different provider. If your trial period is over, it's perfectly acceptable to find a different audiologist to take over your care. Chapter 8 discusses your legal protections in buying hearing aids in more detail.

You are in control of your hearing health. Don't settle for a provider who you feel is not allowing you to have the best hearing possible for you.

CHAPTER 3

What Can I Expect in My First Visits to the Audiologist?

Once you've found an audiologist that you like, I'm sure you'll have a number of questions about the process. Every audiologist office operates just a little bit differently.

Now that I've found an audiologist I'd like to try, what should I do next?

You'll want to call the office and talk to the staff in the front office. Have your questions ready. You may want to ask how many appointments you should expect in the first few weeks and how much time each appointment might take. You may want to ask about basic price ranges to get an idea of a possible budget. And you may want to discuss possible insurance coverage. We'll cover all these topics in this book.

If the office is reluctant to talk about cost, it should be a warning sign. If you call an office and ask, "How much can I reasonably expect to spend on hearing aids, at a minimum, if I come in?" the office should be willing to give you at least the low and high ends of the price range. When a patient calls my office, we make sure to discuss what low-priced, mid-priced, and high-priced hearing devices would cost and what the patient could reasonably expect to get for the additional money. That way, when patients come in they have a good idea of how much to budget and why they might want to climb up in price a little bit.

How much time should I expect to set aside for my appointments?

In general, a hearing test takes about half an hour. That includes some questions about your medical history, the test itself, and talking over the test results. If you already think you have a hearing loss and want to discuss hearing aids, most offices will budget about an hour for your first visit. That will give you time to do the hearing test and talk about your options in hearing devices.

If you feel rushed to make a decision at your first appointment, or if you feel you need more information, by all means make a follow-up appointment. You should never feel pressured to make a decision on day one. You may need time to think about it and talk it over with your family. Don't hesitate to let your audiologist know that you need time and would like to come back and ask follow-up questions on a later day.

Be sure to ask how many appointments you are likely to need in the first couple of months. Getting hearing devices is not an event; it is a process that takes more than one visit. So you'll want to make sure that the audiologist is ready to spend the time needed to make adjustments to the device and to ensure that you're hearing sound that feels the clearest and most comfortable to you.

After the initial hearing test, you will typically need from two to five visits in the next couple of months. These visits are designed to customize the sound of the hearing devices to meet your needs. Be prepared to put in the time to make this experience everything you need it to be. You need to feel comfortable talking to the audiologist and reporting any abrasive sounds or sounds that you're not hearing that you feel you should.

Getting hearing aids is a tailor-made process for each and every patient. Remember, though, that your audiologist can't help you unless you let him or her know what's going on.

Will I know ahead of time what my insurance will cover?

In the past, it was very uncommon for health insurance to cover hearing aids. Today, though, we're definitely seeing a change in the willingness of health insurance companies to cover at least a portion of the cost of hearing aids.

Your audiologist's staff should be able to help you navigate the insurance system. They should be able to tell you, in very clear language, whether your insurance will cover any of the costs. All they will need is the information from your health insurance card to check it out. It's reasonable to ask the office to determine your insurance coverage before your first appointment.

What should I bring along on my first visit to the audiologist?

I would recommend that when you come in for your first visit— the hearing evaluation—you bring a spouse or family member with you. You may be making an expensive life decision, and it always helps to have someone else's input. If that someone else is affected by your hearing loss as well, it's even better to include that person. Communication is a two-way street, and typically the person who is most affected by the hearing loss is a spouse or partner. If you and your partner go in and talk to an audiologist, you may find that your partner noticed your hearing loss long before you did and feels that it is creating more problems in your life than you are aware of. Having that person there with you often will give you the license to go ahead and make a decision to do the right thing for yourself.

You'll also want to bring along your medical records or at least notes on your medical history. At your first visit, your audiologist will probably ask you to fill out a form describing your medical history. This is very important. Most people don't understand why we ask questions about disorders that are seemingly unrelated to hearing loss. We often have people ask, "Why do you want to know if I have high blood pressure, heart disease, or diabetes, or what medications I'm on?" The simple answer is that these things often are related to hearing loss.

As we discussed in chapter 1, many disorders and medications that we would not think would have an effect on us actually affect our entire body system, including our ears. Diabetes doubles your chance of hearing loss, and cardiovascular disease triples your chance.

Insurance coverage and costs involved with hearing aids are covered in chapter 8.

Many medications that we wouldn't think of, including Tylenol and Viagra, increase your chances of hearing loss. It's important for your audiologist to know what medications you take so that when discussing either medical referrals or device options, the audiologist has some idea of how rapidly your hearing loss is likely to progress. Additionally, the audiologist may be able to recommend changes in your medications to discuss with your physician, thereby avoiding medications that might make your existing hearing problems worse.

How will the audiologist test my hearing?

After your audiologist talks to you in depth about your medical history, the next step is usually a hearing test. As we discussed in chapter 2, the hearing test should be done in some type of sound-treated area. This can be a sound-treated room or just a small enclosure within a room, but it should be a quiet area. Sound-treated rooms are generally metal-walled rooms, looking something like a walk-in cooler you would see in a grocery store. Background noise should not bleed through to distract you or cover up the sounds that the audiologist is trying to test.

Once you are in the sound-treated area, you'll be asked to put on headphones. When we're doing a hearing test, we really are looking to test your hearing at its best, not at its worst, which is why it is so important to test in a very quiet environment free from background noise. We want to find out the very softest sounds that you can hear.

The audiologist will usually start by having you listen to detect very soft beeps. Beeps are very reliable and repeatable sounds. If you take a hearing test in my office, I know that the beep portion of the test will match up with the same part of the test if it's done in an office down the street and with tests I might give you later on. This consistency is important for correct diagnosis.

You'll listen to beeps of different pitches. (Think of a pitch as being a note on the piano.) The audiologist will ask you to either raise your hand or press a button every time you hear a beep. The beeps will get softer and softer until the point where you can just barely detect that beep (pitch) 50 percent of the time, which is called your *auditory threshold.* Your auditory threshold is the very softest sound that you can hear. It shows the lowest limits of your hearing when the environment is perfectly quiet.

Once we've determined the softest sounds that you can hear for a wide range of pitches (your auditory threshold), the next step in the hearing test is to find out how well you can understand speech and words. After all, the reason you're looking into hearing aids is most likely that you're not happy with how you hear speech.

We test to determine the softest level of speech that you can hear. During this part of your hearing test, you will be given two-syllable words and asked to repeat them. Every time you get a word right, we'll turn the volume down and give you another word. If you get that one right, we'll turn the volume down again until we find the softest point where you can understand those two-syllable words 50 percent of the time. That's called your *speech reception threshold,* or SRT. In short, your SRT tells you how far away from people you can be and still hear them.

The next type of speech testing that we do in a complete hearing test tells us your *word recognition score,* sometimes called your *speech discrimination score.* We typically have you listen to speech at your most comfortable volume. We'll find out what level sounds loud enough for you—for example, where you would set the volume on the TV if you were listening to speech. At that most comfortable volume, in that perfectly quiet room, we'll give you a list of words to see how many of them you can understand. This will tell us what percentage of speech you understand when everything is perfect—when you're hearing speech at your best with no competing noise.

Another type of test that you may have is a tinnitus evaluation. Tinnitus is any sound that you perceive that is not in the world around you. The most common type of tinnitus is a high-pitched squeal. All of us have left a noisy event and noticed that our ears were ringing. That is temporary tinnitus, but almost 20 percent of the population has that type of sound much of the time. They might have ringing or other noises in their ears all the time, or it may recur intermittently.

Tinnitus can sound like any number of different things: ringing, buzzing, roaring, hissing, thumping, crickets, dinging, or even music. If you have tinnitus that bothers you significantly, your audiologist may also want to do a tinnitus evaluation. Unfortunately, there is no way to put a microphone in your ear and determine how loud your tinnitus is, because it's not a real sound in the vast majority of cases. No one else can hear it. Tinnitus is typically caused by neurologic or biologic activity deep in your ear or in your brain.

If you report tinnitus, you may be asked to complete a questionnaire about the effect the tinnitus is having on your life. You will often be asked to judge how loud the tinnitus is and what pitch it is. This information can often give the audiologist some information about whether a hearing aid or sound therapy device will reduce the impact of tinnitus on your daily life.

When they get a hearing aid, approximately 60 percent of people report that they have some relief from their tinnitus, and some patients even report total relief from their tinnitus while wearing hearing aids.[17] Other devices also are available to give relief from tinnitus and are discussed in chapter 6. The tinnitus evaluation

---

17 S. Kochkin, and R. Tyler, "Tinnitus treatment and the effectiveness of hearing aids: hearing care professional perceptions," *Hearing Review*, 2008; 15 (13): 14–18.

should give you some idea of whether you are one of those people who get some relief.

Your audiologist may also do a speech-in-noise test. Almost everyone with hearing problems reports that their biggest problem is understanding speech in a noisy environment, like in a restaurant. This is not surprising, since a noisy place is also the most difficult listening environment for people with normal hearing. Sometimes, though, we want to figure out if you are having a little difficulty in hearing in noise or if you have a truly debilitating difficulty. In the latter case, it can be useful to see what amount of speech you can hear in the presence of noise.

The most common test puts multi-talker babble in the background—similar to a restaurant or cocktail party. If the test reveals that you have a significant amount of difficulty understanding speech in noise, it indicates that you'll need the most aggressive noise-reduction strategy possible in the hearing device. In extreme cases, supplemental listening devices may be helpful in conjunction with your hearing aids to help overcome the problem of background noise.

Usually, the last part of your hearing evaluation will be bone-conduction testing. This should be part of every diagnostic hearing test. We usually put a small vibrator box behind your ear, where it rests on the bony portion of your skull. Bone conduction is another test that typically uses beeps or tones. We vibrate your skull, which shakes the fluids in your inner ear. You hear it as sound, though, rather than feeling it as a vibration.

When we do bone-conduction testing, we are able to get around the structures of your ear canal, your ear drum, and the bones and muscles of your middle ear, to actually test what your inner ear is hearing directly. Bone-conduction testing helps us find out what part of your ear is experiencing difficulty.

A big difference between the results of your bone-conduction testing and your earphone testing is usually a good sign. It usually means that an ENT physician may be able to improve your hearing loss with either medication or surgery. When there's abnormal bone conduction—when the results of the bone-conduction and earphone tests are very different—the most common disorders that show up are earwax plugging up the ear and ear infections filling the middle ear with fluid. Both of these conditions are easily correctable medically. You may not even need hearing aids to fix the problem.

As a side note, your physician may do a modified bone-conduction test using a tuning fork—holding a tuning fork to your ear and then putting it behind your ear against the bone. If you're able to hear it when it's resting on the bone but not when it's free floating in air, it shows that you have abnormal bone conduction. This is a very basic test, but it can give your doctor enough information to know whether you have a hearing loss, what kind of loss you may have, and whether it is significant enough to warrant having a discussion of possible hearing devices. The tuning fork test is a good first step, but it is really designed to get you in to see your audiologist for a full diagnostic hearing evaluation.

After you have taken the tests, your audiologist should take the time to sit down with you, explain the results, and make sure that you understand what it all means. Most of your test results will be in a graphic form called an audiogram. Your audiogram is so important in your hearing aid success that I've devoted the next chapter, chapter 4, to a discussion of how to read it.

But why do I need a hearing test before getting hearing aids?

Decades ago, hearing aids were simple amplifiers. They'd just make everything louder. They'd make loud sounds louder and soft sounds louder. They'd make low-pitched sounds louder and high-pitched sounds louder. The problem was that those hearing aids were a miserable failure. They didn't take into account an individual's unique hearing loss. If you have normal hearing in the low pitches and terrible hearing in the high pitches, you need a hearing aid that will address those two sounds differently. You want a hearing aid that won't amplify low-pitched sounds at all but will amplify high-pitched sounds very aggressively. As audiologists, we don't know what you need to ask of your hearing aids, though, unless we do a hearing test.

Sometimes patients come into my office and say, "I've resisted having hearing aids for a while because I tried on my husband's hearing aids and they sounded terrible." The patients were well meaning; they thought that they would get an idea of what hearing aids could do for them by trying on any hearing aids. These devices, though, are very similar to eyeglasses. They are fit by prescription and are individualized to your individual hearing loss and your own neurology. You would never try on your friend's eyeglasses, realize that they made you nauseous, and then decide that you must not need eyeglasses.

Similarly, you'd never try someone else's blood pressure medication to see if you needed medication for high blood pressure. You need health care that is individualized to you. You need to try a hearing device that is made for you, not for someone else. You have to try a device that is actually fit to your individual needs to see if it works for you.

In addition, most states require by law that you have a hearing test prior to getting hearing aids. The hearing test must be up to date as well. In my home state, you're required to have a hearing test within six months of ordering hearing aids. This is mainly for your safety. We are not just looking at whether hearing aids are appropriate for you. We're also finding out whether any medical treatment might be necessary. If an audiologist's testing raises any medical red flags whatsoever, we require you to see an ear, nose, and throat physician prior to considering hearing aids. If there's a way to fix your hearing problem through medication or surgery, it is almost always preferable to getting hearing devices. So we want to rule that option out for you, and the only way to do that is with a hearing test.

Please take the time to read chapter 4 before your hearing test. You'll find your visit to the audiologist much more interesting and helpful if you know a little about the tests you'll have ahead of time.

What will happen after my hearing test?

Once you know the results of your hearing test, what you really want to know, of course, is what can be done about any problems that showed up. You waited a long time before making the appointment to go in and talk to the audiologist; you already know you have difficulty understanding speech. What you want to know is how to proceed.

At this point, your audiologist should be able to give you a good idea about the chances of your hearing loss being medically corrected. There are a number of medical red flags that always require a referral from an audiologist to an ear, nose, and throat doctor. Your audiologist will be able to determine whether an ear, nose, and throat doctor has a reasonable chance of treating your hearing problem.

If it looks like your hearing loss is permanent, though, the audiologist will almost certainly start discussing hearing devices as a treatment option. You should expect to talk with the audiologist about different styles of hearing aids, different costs of hearing aids, and how the hearing aids will perform in different listening environments. Your audiologist should let you know what performance and level of success you will get if you decide to spend more or less money.

Your audiologist should explain the pros and cons of each device and help you figure out what device is right for you. You may even have the chance to listen to a device in the office. Ask the audiologist to program up a device to give you some idea about what it would sound like. Not all offices are equipped to do this, but if the office is able to demonstrate a hearing device, it gives you a massive amount of information before you make the decision on whether to buy a hearing device or not. You will know immediately whether things sound clearer, whether they sound more comfortable, and whether speech is easier to understand.

Once you've had your hearing test, talked about your device options, and settled on a budget, your audiologist can order a device for you for a trial period. Depending on what device you have chosen and how severe your hearing loss is, you may or may not need to have an impression taken of the shape of your ear.

An ear impression is a simple and painless process. When we need to custom-make the shape of a hearing aid to fit the ear tightly, which is done more frequently for severe hearing losses, it takes about five minutes. We place a small sponge into the ear canal and then fill the ear with a putty. The putty hardens up in about five minutes, and when we remove it we have a casting of the exact shape of the inside of the ear. We then use this to create a hearing aid that fits comfortably with little risk of falling out, even during physical activity.

What will I do at my hearing aid fitting visit?

On your next visit, the audiologist will program your hearing device for you and begin to teach you how to use it. This visit is called a *hearing aid fitting.*

Be patient with yourself at this visit. You're going to be asked to learn a lot of new skills, the most challenging of which is putting something into your ear. It doesn't sound that difficult, but ever since you were a child you've been told not to stick anything smaller than your elbow in your ear. Now somebody is going to tell you to do just that. Realize that things will feel a little clumsy for the first few days but that it all gets better with practice.

How can I tell if my hearing aids are working well?

Once you've learned the basics of how to operate your hearing aids, you'll have the opportunity to go out and try them in the real world. Your audiologist will suggest that you use your new hearing devices for one to two weeks and then check back in to discuss how things went.

It's very easy to try out a hearing aid in a medical office and think that things sound wonderful. However, I don't think I've ever had a patient come in and tell me, "I want a hearing aid because I want to hear better in your office, Eric." Most people want to hear better in their home, in restaurants, and in the workplace. It's absolutely essential that you take this device out and put it to the test in your real world.

During these first few days of hearing aid use, be sure to keep a list of things that you have really liked and things that you'd like to improve. Keep notes to remind yourself what to tell the audiologist. If there's something specific that's giving you problems, be as specific as possible. For example, you might tell the audiologist, "I generally do pretty well, but I can't hear my wife when she's more than ten feet away." That type of information is absolutely essential to help the audiologist make adjustments so that you can be a successful hearing aid user.

I love when a patient comes in and says, "I'm doing great, but when I rustle the newspaper, it sounds like firecrackers." When somebody is that specific, we can make massive improvements in the sound quality right away. Don't ever feel like you are complaining or being a burden to your audiologist. Audiologists are here for you; you're not here for them. As an audiologist, the worst thing I ever hear from a patient is that they've been leaving their hearing aid in a drawer. If there's something that's bugging you, go in and talk about it. It's your audiologist's job to fix it. You are in charge.

CHAPTER 4

Do I Even Need Hearing Aids? Understanding Hearing Tests

E arly in my career, a woman who I'll call Nancy visited my office for a hearing test. Her children had become alarmed about her hearing, to the point where they didn't want her driving anymore because they didn't feel it was safe. She couldn't hear emergency sirens coming up behind her; she couldn't hear traffic around her. Her family was concerned that she wasn't safe on the road.

The bigger problem, though, was that Nancy didn't believe that she had a hearing loss. She didn't understand that it was time to seek help. When I saw her for her hearing test, she had a severe hearing loss. She could hardly hear any speech at a conversational level. Everyone around her had to speak up or even shout for her to hear them.

In my office, she went into the testing room, and we completed the tests. When she came out of the soundproof area, she informed me that she had done perfectly on the hearing test—that she had heard every beep that I presented to her and had pressed the button every time she heard the beep. The problem was that she didn't know what she didn't hear. She was correct that every time she heard the beep she pressed the button, but she didn't hear approximately 70 percent of the sounds at all. She had no idea they were even occurring.

I then gave Nancy a trial set of hearing aids and presented her with a list of words at a normal conversational level. With the hearing aids on, she understood 80 percent of the words. With the hearing aids off, she understood 0 percent. But she still insisted that she did not need hearing aids. She literally could not register that she was doing better with the hearing aids on.

The fact is that we do not know what we do not hear. We assume that our hearing is perfect because we do hear a portion of speech. The only way to truly know whether you have a hearing loss that affects your speech understanding is to go in and get your hearing tested. Hearing loss isn't only about hearing. It is also about understanding.

In this chapter we talk a lot about a test result called an audiogram. It is my hope that as you learn what this test result means, you'll be better able to have a conversation with your audiologist about whether it is the right time for you to consider hearing aids.

How does my audiologist use my audiogram to find out about my hearing?

As we discussed in chapter 3, your audiologist will test your hearing while you are in a soundproof booth. The results will be plotted on a graph called an *audiogram*, which the audiologist uses to get a good deal of information about your particular hearing loss.

Your hearing test reveals several things that can be incredibly helpful in understanding what sort of hearing loss you have and how much benefit you'll get from hearing aids. You'll remember from chapter 3 that your audiologist will determine your auditory threshold, speech reception threshold, and word recognition score. We'll go through each of these here and learn how to interpret your audiogram to see how you fared in each area, what that tells about the kind of hearing loss you have, and the kind of hearing aid that will thus work best for you. We'll also learn what your bone-conduction test reveals.

What does my auditory threshold mean to me?

When we talk about hearing loss, certain categories describe how severe the loss is. We say a person's hearing is normal or that the hearing loss is mild, moderate, severe, or profound, in order of worsening hearing. Your audiologist will use an audiogram to determine the severity of your hearing loss for various pitches by determining your auditory threshold.

The audiologist will first ask you to listen to beeps of different pitches. (Again, think of a pitch as a particular note on a piano.) As described in chapter 3, the beeps will be made softer and softer until the point where you can just barely detect a particular beep 50 percent of the time. This is your auditory threshold for that pitch. (Remember, your auditory threshold is the very softest sounds that you can hear.) It shows the limits of your hearing in a perfectly quiet environment.

The audiologist will plot the loudness for each beep (or tone) on an audiogram. You will be tested for very deep, bass tones and for very high, shrill, squeaky tones to find the softest sounds that you can hear for a wide range of pitches. We select those particular pitches because they are the most important pitches for understanding speech. In general, the low-pitched, bass sounds that we test correspond very well to vowels. They also correspond very well to nasal consonants like *m, n,* and *ng.* The high-pitched sounds, in contrast, tend to correspond very well to breathy consonants, particularly those produced right in the front of the mouth at the lips and teeth. Sounds like *s, f, t,* and *th* tend to correspond with the highest-pitched sounds we test.

By measuring the softest sounds you can hear at all the different pitches, we can reliably predict what speech sounds you can and cannot hear. That tells us what kind of an effect the hearing loss is likely to have on your daily life.

For example, if you can't hear any of the speech sounds, it's easy to predict how that will affect your daily life: you are going to feel like you're just not hearing anything. Most people with hearing loss, though, have relatively good hearing in the low pitches but significant hearing loss in the high pitches. If that's your case, the hearing test will tell us that you typically will hear people but not understand what they're saying. This is a very different problem to solve than when a patient just can't hear anything.

Take a look at this sample audiogram. The audiologist has plotted the patient's threshold for each pitch (the softest level of sound that allows the patient to just barely detect the pitch) on the graph. The "o" symbols represent thresholds for the right ear, and the "x" symbols represent thresholds for the left ear. If you were able to hear very soft sounds, your thresholds would be located at the top of the graph. The lower your marks fall on the graph, the louder that the sounds have to be for you to hear them. The numbers on the left side of the audiogram are a measure of loudness or intensity. The numbers refer to decibels (abbreviated dB). Larger numbers indicate louder sounds. A 100 dB sound is much, much louder than a 20 dB sound. You are able to hear only that part of the speech area that falls below your thresholds on the audiogram.

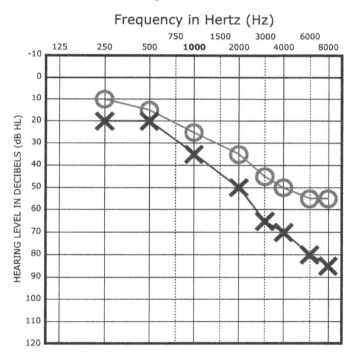

A simple audiogram with air conduction results only. Note that the right ear, circle marks, fall higher on the page indicating better hearing than the left ear, marked by the X's.

If you look at the audiogram, you will see where on the graph each kind of hearing loss falls. In general, if your auditory threshold is between 0 and 20 dB, your hearing is categorized as normal. If your hearing falls between 21 and 40 dB, it's categorized as mild hearing loss. Moderate hearing loss generally falls between 41 and

70 dB. Severe hearing loss falls between 71 and 90 dB, and a hearing loss greater than 90 dB is categorized as profound. These different categories can be incredibly important for understanding how your understanding of speech will be affected by hearing aids.

Common Sounds and Their Typical Loudness in dB Sound Pressure Level:

- Jet engines   140
- Shotgun   130
- Rock concert   110–140
- Power saw   110
- Garbage truck   100
- Subway/motorcycle   88
- Lawnmower   85–90
- City traffic   80
- Washing machine   75
- Vacuum cleaner   70
- Normal conversation   50–65
- Refrigerator hum   40
- Whisper   30
- Rustling leaves   20
- Normal breathing   10

A mild hearing loss causes problems understanding speech when the listening environment is not perfect. People with mild hearing loss can usually understand conversation in a quiet room if they are facing the person who is talking. Many people with mild hearing loss find that hearing aids give them that little bit of added help they need to communicate effectively.

Moderate hearing loss causes difficulty understanding speech in many situations. People with moderate hearing loss may always hear that people are talking, but they will often have trouble understanding speech without wearing hearing aids.

Severe hearing loss and profound hearing loss are devastating to speech understanding unless treated with hearing aids. People with this level of hearing loss frequently find hearing aids extremely helpful, but they will always communicate with difficulty, even when wearing the best hearing aids. If the damage to the ears is so profound that hearing aid use is not enough to allow speech understanding, surgically implanted devices may be discussed as an option.

What is the "most important speech area" that is indicated on my audiogram?

When you're looking at your audiogram, it's important to realize that not every speech sound is the same. The sounds fall on different areas of an audiogram: some speech sounds are low pitched (of low frequency) and some are high pitched (of high frequency). Vowels, nasal consonants, and *r* and *l* sounds tend to fall on the left-hand side of the audiogram in the most important speech area. Breathy consonants such as *s, f, t,* and *th* tend to fall on the right-hand side. If you look at the audiogram in the figure, you will see that some of these speech sounds fall above the plotted line—above the x's and o's—and other speech sounds fall below the plotted line.

Audiogram of Familiar Sounds

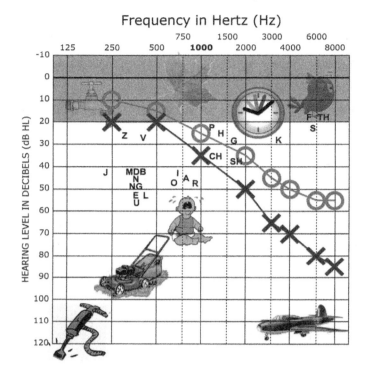

This audiogram shows approximately where some common sounds would fall. Note that any of the sounds that fall below the plotted line can be heard even with this hearing loss. The sounds that fall above the plotted line cannot be heard with this hearing loss.

The audiogram pictured here shows the most common type of hearing loss. This person has relatively good hearing for deep, bass, low-pitched sounds and relatively impaired hearing for shrill, squeaky, high-pitched sounds.

On the left-hand side of the audiogram, the plotted thresholds (the x's and o's) fall further up toward the top of the page. On the right-hand side of the audiogram, the plotted thresholds fall lower on the page. Any of the speech sounds that fall below that plotted line will be audible. Any of the speech sounds that fall above that plotted line will not be heard by this patient.

In this case, patients may think that their hearing is fine. Because they have normal or near normal hearing in the low pitches, they hear vowels just fine. The problem is that they do not understand speech well; note that most of the consonants fall above the plotted line, meaning that the patient cannot hear them. So they will hear one portion of speech but not another portion of speech. When somebody says a sentence such as, "I went to the zoo yesterday," the patient may only hear, "I went o e oo ye-er-ay." When all of the high-pitched consonants that they're not hearing are filtered out, that's what is left.

This is a very typical kind of hearing loss, and this is a very typical experience that people with normal hearing at some pitches and poor hearing at other pitches will have. They will hear, but they will not understand. Still, they will think that their hearing is fine. They hear, "I went o e oo ye-er-ay," so they think that's what the person said. People with this type of a hearing loss often say that it sounds like people are mumbling or not talking clearly. The fact is, though, that they are trying to piece together a jigsaw puzzle with 30 percent of the pieces missing. It's a very difficult thing to do, and that's where hearing devices can help. Hearing aids can actually amplify those high-pitched consonants to a point where you can hear them again, dramatically increasing clarity.

How does my speech reception threshold affect my hearing, and how can my hearing be helped?

As we discussed in chapter 3, once we've determined the softest sounds that you can hear for a wide range of pitches (your auditory threshold), the next step in the hearing test is to find out how well you can understand speech and words. We test to determine the softest level of speech that you can hear—your speech reception threshold or SRT.

We determine your SRT for a couple of reasons. First, we do it to ensure that we're getting an accurate test result. If we look back at your beep testing and average your auditory thresholds at 500 hertz (Hz), 1,000 Hz, and 2,000 Hz, the average of those pitches should be approximately equal to your speech reception threshold. If we see a big difference between your speech reception threshold and the average of your auditory thresholds, we have to suspect that we aren't getting accurate test results. We need to go back and find out why. Perhaps the instructions weren't clear, or there may be a financial reason to exaggerate hearing loss, such as when a lawsuit or disability claim is being made.

The other reason your speech reception threshold is useful is that it tells us how loud speech has to be in order for you to understand it. In short, your speech reception threshold gives us an idea of what your listening distance is—how far away from people you can be and still hear them. Most people are able to understand speech at 20 dB or less. Generally, 0 to 20 dB is considered a normal speech reception threshold. If you have a speech reception threshold between 0 and 20, you should be able to understand speech at a normal conversational level, even all the way down to whispered speech, without much difficulty.

We often use the speech reception threshold to figure out whether it's time for you to get a hearing aid. If we see that your speech reception threshold is normal or near normal, it may be okay for you to wait a little bit before taking the plunge into hearing aids. But if we find that your speech reception threshold is much higher than normal, it's certainly time to get hearing aids. You've waited too long.

A speech reception threshold between 21 and 40 dB is considered a mild hearing loss; this is the point where most people start to notice an effect in their daily lives. At this point, you'll tend to find that your hearing is pretty good if you're face to face with the speaker and in a quiet environment. And even if somebody's back is turned or if they're more than six or eight feet away, as long as the room is quiet you will probably still understand most of what's being said. But at this point you'll start to notice that your primary complaints are that listening to speech in background noise is becoming significantly harder. Restaurants, group meetings, and family gatherings may become more frustrating. And it may be that it's not so much that you don't understand what's being said but that you misunderstand what's being said. This is the point where people start to talk about being afraid that they will respond inappropriately or answer a question that wasn't even asked. When people are at this point, they talk about being afraid of being laughed at in a social setting because they thought one thing was said when actually it was something completely different.

When your speech reception threshold is between 41 and 70 dB, you're categorized as having a moderate hearing loss. When your hearing loss has progressed to this point, you are heavily reliant on optimizing your listening environment. At this point, you really will only be an effective communicator if you're face to face and within six to eight feet of the speaker. People with a moderate hearing loss will say that they cannot hear someone from the next room or cannot understand people whose backs are turned. Background noise makes hearing completely impossible, but hearing is fine as long as it's a face-to-face conversation.

That's the insidious thing about hearing loss. In some listening environments you may do well, but you won't in many others. By the time you have a moderate hearing loss, you are so dependent on trying to find the optimum listening environment that communication during most normal activities is unsuccessful. By the time you have a moderate hearing loss, you absolutely should be investigating the option of hearing devices to improve your situation.

If your speech reception threshold has risen to the point where it's between 71 and 90 dB, you're categorized as having a severe hearing loss. At this point, the hearing loss is impossible to ignore. Without the use of hearing devices, you will be a nonfunctional communicator. People will have to get right up to your ear and raise their voices; they may have to shout. You may be increasingly reliant on lipreading at this point unless you opt to get assistance in the form of hearing devices. Very few people will tolerate a severe hearing loss; most request immediate help.

Once your hearing loss has progressed to the severe level, there are increasing limitations on what the hearing aid can do for you. With severe hearing loss, we tend to see reduced word recognition scores, which reflect how clear the speech that you hear is. Hearing devices will absolutely improve your ability to carry on a conversation, but as we dip down into the severe range of hearing loss, we will find more and more limitations on the ceiling of your performance, such as how effective you can be in challenging environments such as restaurants.

Once your speech reception threshold is greater than 90 dB, you're categorized as having a profound hearing loss. At this point, hearing aids can still provide some benefit, but the clarity of speech will almost always be significantly compromised. Even face-to-face conversation will require the use of visual cues such as facial expressions and gestures. People with profound hearing loss often consider using sign language as a possible supplement to what they're hearing. If your hearing loss has progressed to a profound state, it may be time to go in and talk about surgically implanted devices, such as cochlear implants, if you want to maximize your ability to hear and understand speech. We discuss these devices in greater depth in chapter 6.

Why is my word recognition score so important?

Your audiologist will also give you a word recognition test or speech discrimination test. To determine your score on this test, you'll be asked to listen to speech at your most comfortable volume. We'll find out what sounds loud enough for you—for example, where you would set the volume on the TV if you were listening to speech. At that most comfortable volume for you, in that perfectly quiet room, we'll give you a list of words to see how many of them you can understand. This tells us the percentage of speech you understand when everything is perfect—when you're hearing speech with no competing noise.

Word Recognition						
Word List: NU-6 #1 A				Presentation: Digital		
	dBHL	%	Masking	dBHL	% (aided)	Masking
Right	55 dB	92 %				
Left	70 dB	80 %				

To learn why your word recognition score is so important, let's summarize what we've learned so far. When you have a hearing loss, you typically lose volume and lose clarity. Your speech reception threshold tells you how much volume you have lost. Your word recognition score tells you how much *clarity* you have lost. If you have a hearing loss, you probably do not understand 100 percent of speech even when it's at your most comfortable volume. This happens because you probably have little "blind spots," or distortions, in your hearing. This is important to understand when you get hearing aids. Hearing aids will not just make things louder, and then everything will be perfect. You'll need to have realistic expectations about what hearing aids will actually be able to do for you in the real world.

The word recognition score is the most important predictor for how you'll do with hearing aids in the real world. If I know that in a perfect listening environment, your absolute best word recognition is 60 percent correct, that tells me that no matter what hearing device I give you, you're going to have to use other strategies to understand speech 100 percent of the time. You may have to use your knowledge of grammar and context to understand language; you may have to use facial expressions or watch gestures to help fill in the gaps.

The word recognition score is incredibly important because if I can tell you in advance what the limitations of your hearing aids will be, you will be much, much happier with them. For example, if you know that your maximum word recognition is 60 percent, you won't have unrealistic expectations that a hearing device is going to allow you to understand 100 percent of speech. A hearing device should make things much, much better, but knowing the limitations is very empowering.

In summary, the speech reception threshold tells us how loud speech has to be in order for you to hear it. Word recognition tells us how clear that speech will sound to you once it is loud enough for you to hear it.

Why do you do a
bone-conduction test?

Hearing loss can be conductive hearing loss, sensorineural hearing loss, or mixed hearing loss (a combination of the first two). Chapter 6 describes these kinds of hearing loss in detail.

Essentially, a sensorineural hearing loss is an electrical problem where the vibration of sound is not converted to an electrical signal that your auditory nerve can send to the brain. Sensorineural hearing loss is located deep inside your inner ear or in your auditory nerve or brain.

In contrast, a conductive hearing loss is a mechanical problem where the vibration of sound is being reduced. Conductive hearing losses are normally caused by problems with the ear canal, eardrum, or bones in the middle ear. These structures are much closer to the surface, and surgery or medication is often an option with conductive losses.

A bone-conduction test gives your audiologist a reasonable idea of what type of hearing loss you have. If it turns out that you have conductive hearing loss, your audiologist can refer you for medical treatment and very possibly a cure.

For your bone-conduction test, what you need to know is that conductive hearing loss is a mechanical problem, and it is generally easy to treat medically. In this kind of hearing loss, sound is being damped down. The sound vibrations do not have a clear path through the ear canal or are not getting efficiently passed through the bones of the middle ear. The most common cause is an earwax blockage in the ear canal. If you have a plug in your ear, the vibrations of sound can't get to the eardrum to move the eardrum and the bones of the middle ear. Another common cause of conductive hearing loss is ear infection. In this case, there will be fluid behind the eardrum, and the pressure of that fluid will keep the eardrum from moving normally.

Conductive hearing losses are generally easy to identify and easy to treat medically. If there's a problem that's keeping the structures of the ear from moving normally, a physician can correct that, either through medication or surgery. If the problem is a plug of wax in the ear, a good physician can remove it quickly and easily. If there's fluid behind the eardrum that isn't allowing the eardrum to move normally, that fluid can be drained off. This is accomplished either by curing the infection that's causing it through antibiotics or by putting a small hole in the eardrum to allow the fluid to drain out. Once the fluid is gone, the eardrum will move normally again.

In children, the middle ear is sometimes ventilated to keep fluid from building up. A physician will simply make a small hole in the eardrum and place a tube through it, allowing fluid to drain out as it builds up. This keeps the middle ear dry and, it is hoped, avoids ear infections in the first place.

AUDIOGRAM WITH BONE CONDUCTION

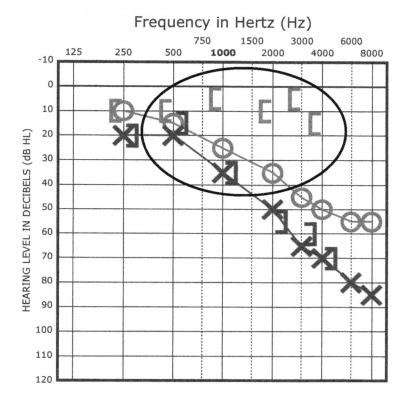

Audiogram with bone conduction. The brackets indicate how well the patient hears through bone conduction. Note that there is a big difference between the air and bone conduction results on this patient's right ear. This means they hear much better through bone conduction and probably have a medically treatable hearing loss.

When we look at the audiogram, we can determine if there's a conductive hearing loss by examining whether there's a difference between air conduction and bone conduction. This can be seen on the audiogram by comparing the x's and o's with the small brackets. The small brackets indicate bone conduction. Bone conduction is determined by putting a small vibrator box behind the ear and shaking or vibrating the skull. This bypasses the mechanical structures of the ear and stimulates the auditory nerve directly.

If your bone-conduction scores (the brackets) are almost identical to your air-conduction scores (the x's and o's), then you do not have a conductive hearing loss. You have sensorineural hearing loss. In this case, hearing devices are the preferred treatment (see chapter 6). But if there's a big difference between the x's and o's on the graph and the brackets on the graph, then we know that you have a conductive hearing loss. In that case, your audiologist will refer you to a medical doctor as part of your treatment. You may still need hearing aids, but medical treatment is the first course of action.

What do blind spots on my audiogram mean for my hearing aid success?

If your hearing loss has progressed to a certain degree, usually into the profound range, it's very possible to have blind spots, often called *cochlear dead regions*, in your hearing. This means that what we measure on the audiogram is not real hearing. What we actually may be measuring is distortion caused at a different pitch than we think we're measuring.

If we see high-pitched hearing loss on the right-hand side of the graph that is worse than 80 dB, we start to suspect that there may be a blind spot in the hearing. What may be happening is that as we're putting enough sound behind a high pitch to stimulate that 80 dB response on the audiogram, we may actually be creating a lower-pitched distortion that you detect—but not as a clear, high-pitched sound.

AUDIOGRAM WITH TYPICAL BLIND SPOT

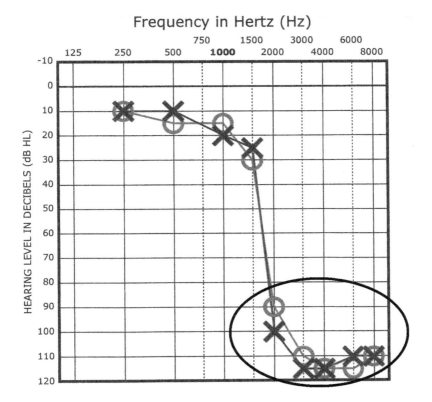

This patient has a very severe or profound hearing loss in the high frequencies. It is very unlikely that these frequencies will ever sound clear to this person. This is, in essence, a blind spot in their hearing.

If you're in a soundproof room taking a hearing test and you have unusual perceptions of a sound—maybe we give you a beep, but it sounds like crickets, static, or chirping but definitely does not sound like a beep—that is a major red flag that you may actually have a blind spot in your hearing, a cochlear dead region. Knowing this is very important in selecting a proper hearing device for you. No matter how loud we make a speech sound, it may not be loud enough for you to hear it at all if you have a blind spot or cochlear dead region. This can have big implications for what type of device we want to proceed with.

If your hearing loss is in the severe or profound range, be sure to ask your audiologist what realistic outcomes you can expect from a hearing device. Also ask if there are any specialty devices that you should consider to maximize your speech understanding. In chapter 6 we discuss hearing devices that can specifically address blind spots in hearing.

CHAPTER 5

Why Is My Hearing Loss Harder to Correct Than a Vision Problem?

W hen patients come to me asking for help with their hearing, most people think of this process as being very similar to getting eyeglasses. It is not.

For example, one patient I'll call Jake came to me with a shoebox full of hearing aids. He had tried five or six sets of hearing aids in recent years, and he had been disappointed by every set. The reason is that fitting hearing aids is very different than fitting eyeglasses. When you're fitting eyeglasses on someone with nearsightedness, all you have to do is focus the image on the eye, and everything is great.

That is because all of the cells that send the visual signal to the brain are still alive and working once light hit them.

Jake actually had a true blind spot in his hearing: there were certain high-pitched sounds that he would never be able to hear no matter how loud we made those sounds. And every attempt at hearing aids in the past had been with very traditional hearing aids, which just tried to make the high-pitched consonants loud enough for him to hear. This was a miserable failure because it was not possible to make him hear these sounds.

With Jake, I had to give up the idea that all I had to do was amplify or focus the sound for him. I had to address the fact that hearing is different than vision—that he in essence had a blind spot in his hearing that we had to deal with. We were able to find devices that could actually shift, or warp, sound so that they brought the high-pitched sounds into a frequency range that he could hear. This allowed him to hear sounds like *s, f,* and *th,* although they would sound different than he remembered before he had a hearing loss.

In addition, we talked about compensatory strategies he could use to allow him to supplement what he wasn't hearing with his vision, with his knowledge of English grammar, and with context. By treating him as a whole patient, rather than just a set of ears, I was able to get Jake to be highly successful with his new hearing aids.

Why do my glasses make things perfectly clear, but I always hear from my friends that hearing aids don't do that?

Hearing aids are not like glasses, because hearing problems are different than the vision problems most people experience. When most people think of vision problems, they think of being either nearsighted or farsighted. Things are just a little out of focus, but the eyes are generally in good health. They don't have blind spots along with their nearsightedness. There's no distortion. There are no holes in the retina. Most people have healthy eyes that can receive light and send that signal up to the brain. All they need to do is get glasses that can focus the light properly.

Unfortunately, that's not the case with hearing loss. With hearing loss, we typically see a loss of the *hair cells* in the inner ear that are responsible for sending a signal up to the brain. Essentially, this means that most people with hearing loss have hundreds of tiny blind spots in their hearing. Even if we make things loud enough or amplified enough, there is just no cell to convert that sound to a language that the brain can understand.

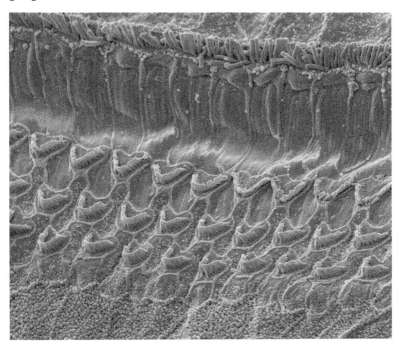

Hair cells. These rows of fibers are from a dissection of the inner ear under an electron microscope. The lower rows of fibers are very orderly and tightly packed together, indicating that they are in good condition. The fibers in the upper row are bent over or broken off, indicating damaged hair cells and impaired hearing.

Hearing loss, then, is much more like nearsightedness plus macular degeneration, a condition that causes blind spots in your eyes. Macular degeneration is a vision problem that often affects older adults, in which some of the sensory cells in the eye are destroyed, causing blind spots. The patient with macular degeneration may have good peripheral vision on the sides but not be able to see anything straight ahead. Say a patient has nearsightedness and a blind spot in the middle of the vision. The eye doctor can correct the nearsightedness with glasses, but he cannot correct the blind spot. In this case, the glasses are more like hearing aids in what they can do: they can correct part of the vision problem but not the whole vision problem.

In hearing loss, you have a loss of outer hair cells, which means that you won't hear soft sounds very well. Sound is not loud enough. You'll need extra volume. In addition to that, you may have a loss of inner hair cells, which means there are tiny blind spots and distortions in your hearing. Hearing is not clear. Hearing aids are designed to correct the loss of outer hair cells by making the softer sounds of speech loud enough for you to hear. What hearing aids cannot correct is the loss of inner hair cells, which affect the clarity of your hearing.

When you lose your hearing, you tend to lose outer hair cells first. These are the cells that are responsible for helping you hear soft sounds. When those go, you lose the ability to hear soft speech or the softer portions of speech, so you may not be able to hear a whisper at all. You will still tend to hear loud sounds just as well as you always did. So although you may not hear a whisper, a shout may still sound painfully loud.

This situation caused big problems with older-technology hearing aids. The hearing aids that were designed in the 1970s and 1980s frequently operated as very simple amplifiers. They would make everything louder. They would make soft sounds louder, and they would make loud sounds louder. That certainly could help sometimes, but the problem was that typically loud sounds became uncomfortable, but soft sounds still weren't loud enough to be audible.

Newer hearing devices can address this issue very effectively through the use of automatic volume control, which we discuss in greater depth in chapter 7. For now, remember that modern hearing aids can deal with your hearing loss just for soft sounds in ways that once weren't possible.

Also, even if you have a substantial loss of inner hair cells, hearing aids should give you a significant benefit. You should never expect hearing aids to get you back to your eighteen-year-old ears—your pre-injury state—but you should expect them to be of significant benefit in most situations. If your inner hair cell loss becomes severe, though, you and your audiologist might need to talk about options in addition to hearing aids.

What happens if I don't treat my hearing loss?

As we discussed in chapter 1, most people put off doing something about their hearing loss as long as possible, and unlike uncorrected vision problems, waiting until a hearing loss is impossible to ignore carries a significant risk.

If you get the correctly prescribed glasses at any time, you'll be able to see clearly right away. In contrast, if you've gone decades without doing anything about your hearing loss, it will probably take time to regain some neurologic and hearing function. When you have a long-term hearing loss, it takes a significant amount of stimulation to regain the brain's ability to understand speech.

If we don't actively use our brain's ability to hear and understand speech, we lose some of that ability over time. We hear with our brain. The ear is just a mechanism to change sound from a physical motion into an electrical signal that can be sent up to your brain. Once that electrical signal goes up the auditory nerve, through the base of your brain, and gets up to the higher language center of your brain, that's when you actually register that sound has been heard. In order for those neurons and cells to remain healthy, they need to have a steady diet of sound. If your auditory neurology does not get stimulation, it can atrophy. It can degenerate. It can become less able to understand the sounds that it receives.

If you have gone a year without treating your hearing loss, it will generally take a month before you get the full benefit of hearing aids. If it's been twenty-four years that you've been ignoring your hearing loss, strap yourself in for about two years during which your hearing will continue to improve as you're wearing the hearing aids. **You should absolutely get benefit from your hearing aids from day one, but it may take a little bit—or a lot—longer to get to your final plateau of performance.**

And remember, there actually is a point of no return. If you ignore your hearing loss long enough, you may never be able to get all of your hearing function back.

How does my hearing change with age?

Most people think that hearing loss is always age related. While it's true that hearing loss is much more likely to occur as you get older, that's primarily due to the fact that you are exposed to more things over time. You are exposed to more toxic substances, high-noise events, and medications. If you're eighty years old, you've had ten times the life experience—and damage to your hearing—as an eight-year-old.

When we go into tribal societies in nonindustrialized nations—say, a tribe in the Sudan—and test the seventy-five-year-olds, we find that their ears hear almost as well as the twenty-five-year-olds in that tribe. They don't have the same degree of age-related hearing loss that we tend to have in our industrialized society.[18]

Ears can remain very healthy late into life. However, there does seem to be an age-related neurologic decline in hearing. A number of studies have shown that between the ages of seventy and seventy-five, our auditory brain stem—an area at the base of the brain that does some of the most basic neurologic processing of sound—loses a number of cells that are responsible for hearing rapid changes in pitch and loudness. Unfortunately, speech is entirely made up of rapid changes in pitch and loudness. This age-related change leads to subtle, hard-to-measure difficulty with hearing when there's background noise as well as difficulty with rapid speech, even in people with normal audiograms.

With this age-related neurologic decline in mind, it's important to understand that if you're in your seventies—even with the best hearing aids that can get you back to hearing soft sounds as well as you did when you were twenty years old—there are some limitations to what the hearing aid can do in background noise. They can certainly make it easier to hear in background noise, but I want to be very careful and caution you that it's important to have realistic expectations and to view your hearing aids as providing *benefits*, not perfection.

---

18 S. Rosen, M. Bergman, D. Plester, A. El-Mofty, and M. H Satti, "Presbycusis study of a relatively noise-free population in the Sudan," *Annals of Otology, Rhinology and Laryngology* 71 (1962): 727–743.

Are there special considerations regarding difficulty in correcting children with hearing loss?

Children with hearing loss are in a special category. The critical period for learning speech and language is from birth to age two. Children who lose their hearing before the age of two, then, will typically experience some delays in acquiring speech and language and will need support from educational professionals.

The most important consideration is whether a child will learn to speak or will learn to communicate through sign language. This sensitive issue is very individual and beyond the scope of this book. At this point, I would just like to say that if your child has a hearing loss prior to the age of two, please consult with deaf educators, speech and language pathologists, and your audiologist in person about what the options are to help maximize the child's ability to communicate either through speech and language or sign language alone.

What can I expect from treatment for my hearing loss?

Very simply, what you should expect from treatment for your hearing loss is *benefit*. You should expect better speech understanding in almost all situations while wearing hearing devices. I'm going to be very careful here and stress that you should expect *benefit* or *improvement*. Hearing devices will not give you perfect hearing 100 percent of the time. You will still have situations where your hearing is not what you want it to be.

I generally tell people to think about it in the following terms: If you put all of your difficulties understanding speech together and then cut them in half, that will be a reasonable expectation from your hearing devices. If you take the number of times you ask for repetitions and reduce it by 50 percent, that is a perfectly realistic expectation of the benefit you'll get from your hearing aids.

Hearing aids will not make your hearing normal and will not completely eliminate your requests for repetition. The reason why is very simple. My personal hearing is better than normal. For most of my life, my hearing has been so good that it's unmeasurable. You can't even plot it on the audiogram. But I *still* ask people to repeat what they've said. With better-than-normal, off-the-chart, unmeasurably good hearing, I still have difficulty sometimes. Therefore, with a hearing loss and hearing aids, you will still have difficulty at times, too.

The most common situation in which people want improvement in hearing is amid background noise, such as at a restaurant or party. An interesting study done a few years back asked a number of people, "How much speech do you think you understand when you're in a cocktail party setting?" Hearing-impaired people who did not use hearing aids said they understood between 15 and 20 percent of speech in that situation. Those with one hearing aid said they understood about 35 percent of speech, and those with two hearing aids said they understood about 65 percent of speech. People with normal hearing said they understood about 70 percent of speech.[19]

So when you choose to get hearing devices it's important to remember that they will not get you back to understanding 100 percent of speech—because no one hears perfectly. Even people next to you at a party with normal hearing feel like they are smiling and nodding and faking it 30 percent of the time. If you're eating out in a

---

19 A. Markrides, "Reaction to binaural hearing aid fitting," Scand Audiol Suppl. 1982; 15: 197–205.

restaurant with your hearing devices and you feel like you're smiling and nodding and faking it only 30 percent of the time, that's a pretty good outcome. That means you're doing about as well as somebody with normal hearing.

What you should find is that when you wear your hearing devices, there's an *improvement.* I suggest that the first week you get your hearing devices, you go out to a restaurant and listen to half of the meal conversation with the hearing aids in and the other half with the hearing aids out. Sit through the salad with the hearing devices on as you talk to your dining companion, then sit through the entrée with the hearing aids out, and you will immediately see whether there's a difference. When people do that, they tend to report things like, "Okay, when I was without the hearing aids, I understood 20 percent of the conversation. With them in, I understood 60 to 70 percent of the conversation." I would definitely call that a successful outcome.

The problem is that we get caught up in wanting 100 percent. We have actually forgotten that "normal" hearing is not perfect hearing. We actually want our hearing aids to get us better-than-normal hearing, which is not realistic.

So it is important to understand that hearing aids are designed to get you as close to normal as you can possibly get. Hearing well in very difficult listening environments, such as hearing somebody when you're in the back seat of the car and they're in the front seat, probably is not a reasonable expectation. Hearing your spouse talking from the next room while you're running water in the sink is probably not a reasonable expectation. However, it certainly is reasonable to expect improvement in almost every listening environment. If you understand 20 percent with the hearing aids out and you understand 70 or 80 percent with the hearing aids in, that's what we're going for.

I have the most trouble understanding my spouse. Why doesn't he just talk more clearly?

One of the most common requests my patients make for their hearing aids is to understand their spouse or partner better: "I can hear other people pretty well, but I can hardly hear my wife or husband at all." Spouse-to-spouse or partner-to-partner communication is different than any other kind of communication.

We have different conversational habits with our family members than we have with anyone else. We cut corners with our spouse that we would never cut with an acquaintance. We would never invite a buddy over to our house, walk out of the room, turn our backs on them, turn on the water, do dishes, and expect to carry on a conversation. But this is completely common between married couples. I'm not trying to place blame here, but it helps to be aware that this is something we do with the people we're around most of the time. We don't take the same care in talking to them that we take with our friends.

When you have normal hearing, you may or may not hear each other well. I guarantee, though, that if you have a hearing loss and you try to carry on a conversation from the next room with the water running, it's not going to work—no matter which hearing aids you bought.

Having said all of that, even though we are sloppier in our communication habits with our spouses, difficulty understanding them can be the first indicator of a hearing loss. Because the communication environment and habits are more difficult, mild hearing losses will be much more obvious when you are communicating with your spouse in the home. If you're feeling like you understand everyone just fine, but not your spouse, that is a major red flag. It's time to go in and have your hearing tested.

CHAPTER 6

What Types of Help for My Hearing Loss Are Available?

T here is a limit to what hearing aids can do. Hearing aids are amplifiers; they are not replacements for the ear.

A patient I'll call Julie came in to see me recently. She was in her fifties and worked in retail. She had a fairly severe hearing loss and already wore hearing aids. She came to me hoping to be able to hear better in those noisy stores, as well as on the phone. She hoped that the newer, high-tech hearing aids might allow her to communicate more effectively. Unfortunately, she had such a severe hearing loss and so much distortion in her ears that no hearing aid I put on her was going to allow her to hear clearly in those situations.

After evaluating her performance with the highest-tech hearing aids on the market, we determined that she needed a different approach. We went through a long counseling session about a device called a cochlear implant, which is a surgical device that we talk about at length later in this chapter as an alternative to hearing aids in cases of severe hearing loss. In this particular case, it made much more sense to refer Julie to a physician for a surgical consultation.

If you have a severe hearing loss, there are many types of treatments that we can talk about. Some of them are hearing aids, some of them are other devices, and some of them are simply education and strategies. Every person is an individual, and there is no one set way an audiologist can help everyone meet their goals. When you talk with your audiologist, you can expect to have a discussion about what your particular goals are and which treatment options, out of all of the ones available, are best for you and why.

As you read in chapter 4, the type of help your audiologist can provide varies according to the type of hearing problem you have.

I have conductive hearing loss. How can this type of hearing loss be treated?

Conductive hearing loss is a mechanical problem in your ear. To put it simply, parts of the ear are not moving. The air molecules in the ear canal may not be moving because of a plug of earwax, and thus they cannot cause the eardrum or bones of the middle ear to move, allowing you to hear. This type of hearing loss is the kind that is most treatable by medical therapies.

If you have a conductive hearing loss, your ear, nose, and throat doctor will be involved every step of the way.

The doctor will try to remove the impediment that is keeping the structures of the ear from vibrating. There may be a plug of earwax that can be removed or an infection that can be cleared up with antibiotics. In some cases, surgery may be used to either drain off fluid from the middle ear or to reconstruct bones that have been broken or degraded.

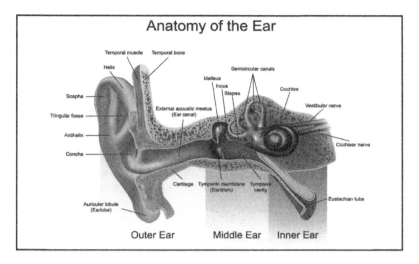

This drawing shows the major structures of the outer, middle, and inner ear.

Conductive hearing loss can be medically corrected most of the time. However, in certain instances the conductive hearing loss will be permanent. In these cases, a couple kinds of hearing devices can help. The first type is a traditional hearing aid. Because the problem with conductive hearing loss is simply that vibrations are being damped down or softened, and a hearing aid makes vibrations louder, or bigger, hearing aids work phenomenally well with conductive hearing loss. Once we make sound loud enough, it typically will be very, very clear. People who have corrected a conductive hearing loss with hearing aids hear very similarly to someone with normal hearing.

There are times, though, when hearing aids do not work well with a conductive hearing loss. A chronic ear infection that causes fluid to drain out of the ear will cause a hearing aid to malfunction. People with certain birth defects may not have a visible ear or ear canal, so sound cannot enter the skull. In these cases, a new type of device called a bone-anchored hearing aid is surgically implanted. It causes the skull to vibrate, which then vibrates the fluids of the middle ear.

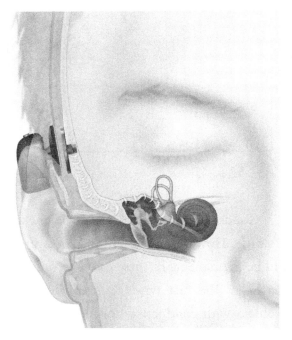

Picture of a bone-anchored hearing aid. Note there is a snap or button embedded in the bone. The box outside the head will vibrate that snap and the skull it is attached to. Those vibrations will shake the fluid in the inner ear allowing the wearer to hear. Picture courtesy of Cochlear Corp.

If I have a sensorineural hearing loss, how can it be treated?

Sensorineural hearing loss is caused by damage to the hair cells in the inner ear or damage to the auditory nerve. The inner ear, or cochlea, changes sound from a mechanical sound to an electrical signal; the auditory nerve carries that electrical signal up to the brain where hearing actually occurs. This damage commonly occurs due to exposure to loud noise, aging, and heredity.

Sensorineural hearing loss is treated with hearing devices, rehabilitation strategies, or both. Hearing devices include hearing aids (including assistive listening devices, personal sound-amplification devices, and tinnitus instruments, all discussed in this chapter, as well as cochlear implants). Rehabilitation strategies might entail lipreading, sign language, and active listening therapy.

Which treatment or combination of treatments that might work best for you will depend on your own particular hearing loss. Your audiologist will discuss the options with you and give you the information you'll need to decide what will help you the most. Since sensorineural hearing loss is so common, the rest of this chapter is devoted to these.

How do hearing aids help with a hearing loss?

For the vast majority of people with sensorineural hearing loss, hearing aids are the most effective kind of treatment available. This is because the first structures in the ear to be damaged are typically the outer hair cells. These are the cells that make sounds loud enough for the brain to interpret. Modern hearing devices selectively amplify soft sounds and don't necessarily amplify loud sounds. They try to replace the function of those cells that are most commonly lost.

With the best possible fitting of hearing aids, you should feel not so much that you're getting a lot of volume or loudness but that you're gaining clarity. The hearing aids should selectively amplify whispered speech while letting shouted speech come through as if it's not amplified at all. The bottom line is that hearing aids should make soft speech audible, moderate speech comfortable, and loud speech tolerable. If we can do that, you're generally going to have good success with your hearing aids.

Are cochlear implants an option for me?

If your hearing loss is in the severe to profound range, there is a diminishing level of return with hearing aids. They may still be a significant help to you in understanding speech, but sometimes a surgically implanted device called a cochlear implant may be a better choice. If your word recognition score has dropped significantly—if at your most comfortable volume you can hear and understand only 30 to 40 percent of words—a cochlear implant may help you.

In a severe to profound hearing loss, decreased clarity occurs because you have lost inner hair cells in your ear. These are the cells that convert sounds to electrical impulses, which travel up to the brain. Once the inner hair cells are damaged or have died off, they don't grow back. This leaves you with tiny blind spots in your hearing. If you have enough deterioration of the inner hair cells, your clarity of speech drops dramatically because the sound is no longer being efficiently transduced into an electrical signal.

A cochlear implant seeks to get around this problem. This is a surgically implanted device. It consists of a wire with around twenty-two to twenty-four electrodes attached to it that is placed inside your inner ear. The wire is wrapped around the end of your auditory nerve, and the electrodes stimulate your auditory nerve electrically. This takes over the function of the inner hair cells. When the auditory nerve is stimulated electrically, that electrical impulse gets sent up to the brain, where it can be interpreted as sound or speech. Even though the stimulation is electrical, your brain can interpret it as sound. Remember, converting sound to electricity is what a healthy inner ear does. The cochlear implant attempts to take over that process when the inner ear has been catastrophically damaged.

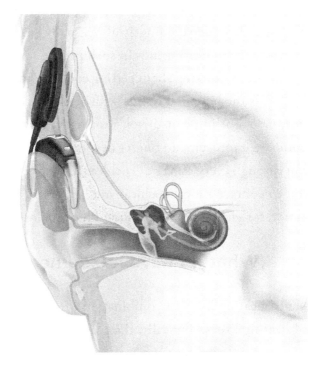

Picture of cochlear implant. Here you can see that there are two components. The sound processor is worn over the ear but communicates with another piece. The internal electrode array is implanted under the skin, and electrodes are inserted into the inner ear. The cochlear implant is a prosthetic inner ear, not a hearing aid. Picture courtesy of Cochlear Corp.

It's important to note that cochlear implants are not going to make you hear like you did with your eighteen-year-old ears. After all, instead of using fifteen thousand cells in your ear, they use twenty-five electrodes to try to give you information about speech.

Patients often tell us that speech through a cochlear implant can sound cartoonish or robotic—almost like people are talking like Mickey Mouse or Donald Duck. Usually, people report that voices they're familiar with usually sound fairly natural, but new voices may not. However, even though speech may not sound clear or natural with cochlear implants, it typically sounds clearer than what hearing aids can produce with a severe to profound sensorineural hearing loss. And speech understanding is also usually improved with cochlear implants versus hearing aids in such people.

If you're thinking about getting cochlear implants, it is important to discuss the potential results with a cochlear implant team in your area. Cochlear implants involve major surgery. They can provide an immense improvement, but it's beyond the scope of this book to take you through every aspect of cochlear implants. So again, I encourage you to contact a local cochlear implant team. They may be a viable option for your severe to profound hearing loss.

What if I have mixed hearing loss?

Mixed hearing loss is a combination of conductive and sensorineural hearing losses. Typically, the conductive portion of your hearing loss can be treated by a medical doctor. The sensorineural portion is treated by an audiologist.

My hearing aids are not enough when I'm watching television or listening to a lecture. Can anything help?

Not everyone gets as much benefit from hearing aids or cochlear implants as they would like. The most common complaints are "I have difficulty understanding in background noise," "I have difficulty understanding speech at a distance," and "I can't understand television very well."

Sometimes technology in addition to hearing aids can be of great help. *Assistive listening devices* connect your hearing aid directly to the sound source you want to listen to. For instance, many people come into my office and say, "I need better clarity for the television. I'm turning the volume up louder than my family would like."

In this case, we can put a wireless transmitter on the television to send the sound from the TV directly to your hearing aids. That allows you to turn your hearing aids into wireless headphones, essentially plugging your hearing aids directly into the TV. This process overcomes the loss of clarity that occurs as sound travels through the air from a distance—from the television to your hearing aids. It also overcomes any problems with background noise in the room. When you patch your hearing aid directly into the television, the only thing you're amplifying is the television. And that can make a massive difference in the clarity of the sound you hear.

We can also use this same idea in a lecture or classroom setting. If you're having difficulty hearing speech at a distance, you could have the lecturer wear a small wireless transmitter mic clipped onto his or her collar to transmit directly to you wherever you are in the audience.

This process may sound a bit cumbersome because you do have to ask the lecturer to wear a transmitter mic. However, it can be an amazing benefit for people who struggle with large lecture settings. The same approach can be used in colleges, high schools, and even churches. Most churches have some sort of sound system already installed, and there may be a way to patch your hearing aids into that existing sound system. Your audiologist can tell you what to do.

Is there any way I can hear better on my cell phone?

Cell phones are frequently a source of complaints with hearing aids. Again, assistive listening devices can help.

Believe it or not, the best-sounding telephones we've ever had in this country were probably designed in the 1950s. They were robust and heavy. The loudspeakers were driven by a high-quality magnet and powered by electricity. All of these things contributed to a better sound quality. Today, the emphasis is on making phones smaller and more portable, and we've sacrificed some sound quality in the process. It's common for people to say, "I hear well on my landline phone, but I don't hear well on my cell phone."

A number of assistive listening devices can allow your cell phone to wirelessly transmit the phone call to your hearing aids with a much higher quality. These devices usually employ a transmission medium called Bluetooth, which is built into most modern cell phones.

In addition, the phone call can be sent to both ears at once, if you're wearing two hearing aids. This allows you to use the best parts of hearing in both ears to interpret the phone call, which can be a massive improvement for many patients. Many people with hearing aids understand 40 to 50 percent of speech in each ear individually—but they understand 80 to 90 percent of speech when they use both ears together. These specialized devices are typically designed for a specific brand of hearing aid, so each manufacturer has its own version. Your audiologist should be well versed in helping you pick the best cell phone assistive listening device for your needs.

I saw something called a personal sound amplification device at the drugstore. Is this something worth looking into?

At a pharmacy or electronics store, you may have seen a display for *personal sound amplification devices* or PSAs. Patients ask me about them fairly frequently. You need to know that these devices are not actually hearing aids; they are simple amplifiers that are sold over the counter without a doctor's prescription. If you read the package, you'll note a disclaimer saying that they're not designed for hearing loss. However, all of the large text on the package will certainly lead you to the conclusion that they can help with a hearing loss.

These simple amplifiers make soft sounds louder, and they make loud sounds louder. They are not acoustically tuned for your particular hearing loss. You will recognize a personal sound amplification device because it is typically priced anywhere from $20 to $200, whereas hearing aids typically are priced close to $1,000 or more. In addition, because they're not designed for hearing loss, PSAs are not subject to the same laws as hearing aids. And because they're not fit to prescription, they can be sold over the counter.

A good rule of thumb is that if you don't have to have a hearing test and you don't have to have a professional involved to look in your ear and tell you what your problem is, what you are buying is not an actual hearing aid. And it probably is not going to give you the results that you really need.

Is there something that can help me with my tinnitus?

If you have tinnitus, you know how bothersome it is. Tinnitus is any sound that you can hear that is not actually in the world around you. Tinnitus can sound like buzzing, roaring, ringing, hissing, or thumping.

If you don't need hearing aids, a tinnitus device may help. This device is designed for people with ringing or other noises in their ears. It won't usually get rid of the tinnitus, but it is designed to make the ringing or other noises in your ear less annoying. It accomplishes this by running interference with another sound. If your tinnitus sounds very abrasive, like fingernails on a chalkboard, we may be able to replace it with a pleasant sound like ocean waves or wind chimes. There are a number of these sound therapy strategies on the market, and your audiologist should be able to help you decide which device would be best for you and then tune the sound therapy to provide the maximum benefit.

If you have tinnitus and also need hearing aids, the hearing aids alone may be enough to interrupt tinnitus and provide relief. However, you also might want to consider getting a combination hearing aid / tinnitus sound therapy device, usually called a *tinnitus instrument*. These devices act as hearing aids but also can be programmed to put out a sound therapy—to disrupt the tinnitus when you want it to. Such devices do not get rid of the tinnitus but may cover it up with a second sound that is more pleasant or can distract you from the tinnitus. This allows your brain to stop focusing on the tinnitus and to stop viewing it as a threat or a danger, which in turn allows you to push the tinnitus into your subconscious.

A tiny minority of tinnitus sufferers find their tinnitus so disturbing that it interrupts sleep, causes depression and anxiety, and in extremely rare cases even causes suicidal thoughts. It is interesting to note that Vincent van Gogh had a disease that caused chronic tinnitus, which was very disturbing to him. Some people postulate that he cut off his ear in an effort to make the tinnitus stop.

A number of therapies and medications can help with the mental health side of tinnitus. If you are having depression or thoughts of harming yourself, please bring this to the attention of your physician, your mental health professional, and your audiologist as soon as possible. Help is available.

Would learning to lip-read help me?

Lipreading used to be a more common rehabilitation technique for people with severe or profound hearing loss than it is today. Unfortunately, lipreading is not a particularly effective way of communicating. Only 20 to 30 percent of the speech sounds are visible on the face. Most of these sounds are produced back in the throat, where the viewer simply cannot see what's going on. Even for the speech sounds that are visible, many will look identical. For instance, *p, b,* and *m* all look exactly the same on the face.

I used to work in a clinic where we would take people through a sixteen-week course in lipreading. They would meet multiple times a week and end up with approximately forty-five hours of training. We found that their ability to lip-read went up maybe 1 to 2 percent. This is simply not an effective therapy for most people.

How about sign language? Who can benefit from learning to use it?

Sign language can be an extremely effective mode of communication for patients who cannot communicate verbally even with the best hearing devices or surgeries or who simply want to be a part of the Deaf culture and the Deaf community. Be aware, though, that learning sign language really is learning a whole new language with its own grammar, vocabulary, and culture.

Most people who suffer hearing loss later in life are not terribly successful with sign language for the simple reason that no one else in their life speaks it. It usually is not helpful in connecting you with your existing community of oral communicators.

Children, however, often benefit greatly from learning sign language. Teaching sign language, either with or without oral communication skills, usually gives young hearing-impaired children faster access to language than hearing alone can.

If you have a young child with a hearing loss, consult with a deaf educator, a speech-language pathologist, and an audiologist about which communication mode may be best for your child. The best route may be oral education alone, sign language alone, or a combination of sign language and oral communication, which is called *total communication*. The decision is a very individual one that should be up to the parents. The goal of this book is only to familiarize you with the concept of deaf education and to encourage you, particularly if you have a child younger than two with a hearing impairment, to seek out professionals in your area to get firsthand advice about what is best for your child.

Is there any benefit to active-listening therapy?

An increasing number of computer-based therapy programs are being marketed to use what's called *neuroplasticity*, or the ability of the brain to restructure itself with experience. These therapies can be used to help improve memory, to help you with problem solving, or to even help hold off dementia or Alzheimer's. We're also seeing neuroplasticity therapies that are said to help with listening tasks.

A number of computer-based programs use guided and focused listening tasks to try to optimize your neurologic ability to interpret sound. The idea is that most people put off getting hearing devices for years, allowing their brains to become less specialized for hearing sounds because of disuse. These programs are supposed to be like physical therapy for your brain; if you can retrain your brain to make better use of sounds, your speech understanding will go up.

This all sounds good on paper, and it may pan out in the real world. Currently, though, there is not in my opinion enough data to show that active-listening therapies create a real-world benefit. If your audiologist offers an active-listening therapy that is low cost, by all means try it to see if you feel it's a benefit.

I would also suggest that if you are considering an active-listening therapy that costs thousands of dollars, ask the prescribing professional for data that proves that the therapy is effective. You as the consumer should be comfortable in requesting solid information on your prognosis if you undergo this therapy.

I don't like my hearing aids. Is there any point in taking them to a new audiologist to see if something can be done to allow me to hear better?

As an audiologist, I spend a good deal of time working with people who have spent a good deal of money elsewhere on what could be considered failed hearing aid fittings. Many of these patients did not make an informed or smart choice about who they did business with. Instead of getting health care, they wound up buying a device that was improperly set for them.

You may have spent thousands of dollars on hearing aids that you cannot wear. You may have found that there's too much background noise or that you sound like you're talking in a barrel or that things just aren't clear. If this is the case, do not despair. Hearing aids frequently can be reprogrammed or readjusted by another provider to better meet your needs.

A hearing aid is much more than just a device. When you purchase hearing aids, what you're really purchasing is the provider's expertise on how to program and set these devices to best process sounds for your individual needs.

When your audiologist gets hearing aids from the manufacturer, they don't come preset for you. They can be programmed to fit a number of different levels of hearing loss—anywhere from mild

100

all the way up to severe. If the professional that you're dealing with doesn't know how to program those hearing aids, you can wind up with wildly inappropriate sound being pumped out of them and into your ears.

If a professional ever tells you, "Just get used to it. You just need to wear them more," you're probably dealing with a professional who doesn't know how to adjust the hearing aids well. There should be a give-and-take in setting your hearing aids.

It's normal to expect three or four follow-up visits after the initial fitting with a hearing device to make it sound as good as possible for you. The professional will probably try to stretch your comfort zone and maybe push you to accept a little bit more sound than you're 100 percent comfortable with initially. The idea is that your brain and your ears will become accustomed to that sound.

But if you're seven or eight appointments in and you're still not satisfied, it's time to find someone else to help you with your hearing aids. If your hearing aids still sound terrible several months into wearing them, pick up the phone and call someone else. Often all it takes is a new set of eyes—maybe a new skill set—to look at how the hearing aids are programmed, listen to your particular concerns, and make a compromise so that the hearing aid can deliver more of what you're hoping for. You should never have hearing devices sitting in a drawer.

A lot of people assume that once they have a pair of hearing aids, another audiologist would not be willing to program or adjust those hearing aids for them. They worry that it would be rude or in bad form to switch to another health-care provider.

Your audiologist is here for you. If you are not feeling that you're clicking well with an audiologist, or that your concerns are not being addressed well, it is up to you to find somebody who addresses your problems better and switch to that provider. As health-care professionals, we know that none of us is going to be the perfect fit for everyone; we all have unique personalities and skill sets. I might refer a patient to another clinic across town if I feel I'm not the best fit, and other clinics will refer patients to me if I have something that I can offer that they cannot. This is not personal. This is about getting you to the health care that you need.

You do need to be prepared for the fact that asking an audiologist to spend hours of appointment time with you to program hearing aids that you purchased elsewhere will likely carry a cost. You should not expect an audiologist to spend hours adjusting your hearing aids and not receive a bill. You purchased the hearing aids from somebody who could not complete the job to your satisfaction and you paid them money, but the next audiologist along the way should still be compensated. Audiologists commonly have an hourly charge to reprogram hearing aids that were purchased elsewhere.

The reprogramming fee, though, is typically a fraction of the cost of buying new hearing aids. So if you have hearing aids that you are dissatisfied with and that are sitting in the drawer, you owe it to yourself to see if there's anything that can be done so that they work for you. The cost to readjust the hearing aids will typically be well worth it in the end.

CHAPTER 7

How Do Hearing Aids Work for Me?

Choosing the right type of hearing aid is incredibly important. A patient who I'll call Matthew came to me who had been fit with the smallest hearing aids on the market. They were completely in the ear canal. The reason he was fitted with them is that he went to his hearing aid dealer and said he didn't want his hearing aids to be noticed. The hearing aid dealer was happy to accommodate him because that particular office had its highest profit margin on tiny, completely-in-the-canal hearing aids.

Unfortunately, this type of hearing aid was a disastrous choice for Matthew. His particular hearing loss was completely inappropriate for this kind of hearing aid. As soon as he put the hearing aids in his ears, he felt like he was talking with his head in a barrel or with his ears plugged up with earplugs. Needless to say, he immediately stopped wearing them. He had spent over $7,000 on those hearing aids, and they were sitting in a drawer.

When he came to me, we first talked about what he thought he wanted. Then we talked about the different types of hearing aids he could have and what would actually meet his needs.

In the end, we selected an open-fit hearing aid, which is a type of behind-the-ear hearing aid. It leaves the ear canal wide open, allowing the wearer's voice to sound much more natural. It also improved Matthew's speech understanding and background noise in places like restaurants.

If Matthew had had the knowledge that you are getting by reading this book, he would have been able to go in and effectively communicate his problems to his hearing aid dealer in the first place. The end result would have been less frustration and more success, and he would have saved a lot of money.

This chapter provides an overview of the main types of hearing aids. We also discuss many of the specific features that may make one particular hearing aid more effective than another and why you might choose an in-the-ear hearing aid versus a small behind-the-ear hearing aid. This information is detailed and changes rapidly as technology improves. You will certainly want to follow up with your audiologist regarding specific features when considering new hearing aids.

How does modern technology create better hearing aids and make my life better?

Hearing aids used to be simple amplifiers. They simply made every sound louder. They could not be tuned effectively to your particular type of hearing loss.

Modern hearing aids, though, are by prescription. They are fitted to your exact hearing loss and target the types of sounds that you don't hear. Most commonly, those are soft, high-pitched sounds.

What you probably need in hearing aids is not simply amplification; you need amplification plus volume control. When you're missing soft, high-pitched sounds, you need amplification for the softer portions of speech (*s, f,* and *th*) but not for the louder portions of speech. When effectively fitted, modern hearing devices take this into account. They meet your individual needs and selectively amplify just the sounds that you're missing. The end result is that with a modern hearing device, you should feel not so much that things are louder but that things are clearer. This means you'll be more satisfied.

How does the audiologist know what I need?

When we fit modern hearing devices, we use what's called a prescription formula—basically a mathematical formula that tells us how much amplification you need at each different pitch for best speech understanding. We begin with the results of your hearing test or audiogram (see chapter 4). If you have normal hearing for deep, bass sounds, we don't give you any additional power for those normal hearing pitches. If you have a substantial hearing loss at a particular pitch, we try to give you amplification equal to approximately half of your hearing loss back at that pitch.

This may sound surprising. Hearing aids do not give you 100 percent of your hearing loss back. If you have a 50 dB hearing loss, we give you less than 50 dB of amplification. Most people think that hearing aids should bring your hearing back to fully normal. If we gave you access to all the sounds that you've been missing, you would be overwhelmed. You would feel like you were inundated with background noise and that you couldn't hear through it at all. By bringing back approximately half your hearing loss in terms of amplification, we're able to present you with the most important speech sounds without overloading you with background noise.

It's important to remember that hearing aids don't get you back to normal, but they should get you a good deal closer than you were without them.

What choices do I have for shapes and styles of hearing aids?

One of the things that people think about most when they're considering hearing aids is cosmetics: How small can the hearing aid be? How invisible can it be?

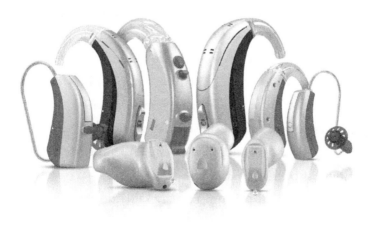

Pictures of various styles of hearing aids including behind-the-ear, receiver-in-the-canal, and custom-shaped, in-the-canal hearing aids. Photo courtesy of Widex.

Although cosmetics are important, it's even *more* important to get hearing aids that perform well—that help you understand speech. After all, that's why you are going to the audiologist.

There are three main styles of hearing aids to consider: behind-the-ear, in-the-ear, and completely-in-the-canal hearing aids.

A behind-the-ear, or BTE, hearing aid has its electronics outside and, obviously, behind the ear, and a small tube or wire goes down into the ear canal to direct sound to the eardrum. This kind of hearing aid can be very large if the hearing loss is severe to profound, or it can be so small it is almost invisible in people with mild hearing loss—and anywhere in between.

Today, approximately 85 percent of people prefer some type of BTE (behind-the-ear) device (sometimes also referred to as mBTE for mini behind-the-ear, RIC for receiver-in-the-canal, RITE for receiver-in-the-ear, or mRITE for mini receiver-in-the-ear).

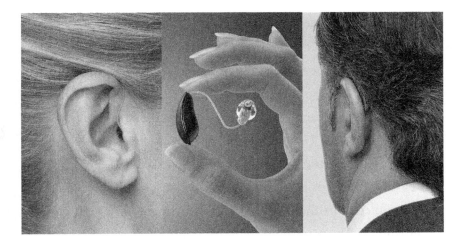

Picture of mRITE hearing aid from several angles. Modern over-the-ear hearing aids can be much more cosmetically appealing than people expect. In most cases, they look much better than in-the-ear or in-the-canal hearing aids.

Even though this style is more noticeable than the smallest completely-in-the-canal styles, it often sounds more natural. By moving the electronics out of the ear, we are able to open up a large tunnel through the earpiece in the ear canal. This allows your own voice to sound more natural to you. People with in-the-ear hearing aids sometimes say it sounds like they are talking into a barrel. This is not a problem with behind-the-ear devices.

In addition, BTE hearing aids are typically as comfortable, if not more comfortable, than the in-the-ear styles we'll discuss next. Because the bulk of the electronics are not in the ear canal, there is less physical mass and pressure inside the ear.

The second type of hearing aids—"in-the-ear" or ITE hearing aids, sometimes called custom-made hearing aids—fill up most of the ear canal. These gained popularity in the 1970s and 1980s, when BTE hearing aids were extremely large, heavy, and uncomfortable. However, the ITE style made wearers' voices sound quite distorted to themselves when they talked, like talking with a bad cold or hearing a tape recording of themselves talking.

Then, in the 1980s, President Ronald Reagan came out of the closet and told everyone that he had a hearing loss and wore hearing aids. He wore a type of hearing aid called the "in-the-canal" hearing aid or ITC hearing aid. Once Reagan let everyone know that even the president of the United States could have a hearing loss and be effective, everyone asked their audiologist for the president's hearing aid. ITC hearing aids became very popular.

Completely-in-the-canal or CIC hearing aids are tiny—the closet thing we have to invisible hearing aids, even smaller than the ITC style that President Reagan wore. They generally sit entirely in the ear canal. If you look closely inside a wearer's ear, you will probably find the hearing aid, but they are very difficult to see. From a cosmetic standpoint, a CIC hearing aid is the best option.

These hearing aids, however, have some significant negatives. Because they block the ear canal, they will make your own voice sound very distorted to you; it will sound like you have a terrible head cold. To get an idea of what this would sound like, put your fingers in your ears as you're reading this, and say a few words. You will immediately know what I'm talking about when I tell you that your own voice will sound distorted with a CIC hearing aid.

The other negative is that some of the newest hearing aid technologies are not available in the CIC devices, so you often lose some performance, particularly in noisy environments, by stressing cosmetics instead of technology. One of the most important technologies that are not included in CIC devices are directional microphones to improve hearing in background noise, which will be discussed later in this chapter. The reason they cannot be included in CIC devices is that the two microphones usually need to be at least six millimeters apart to help you focus more on what's in front of you and less on what's behind you. A CIC hearing aid does not have enough room to put those microphones in that configuration. So if you would like the best possible hearing in moderate amounts of noise, such as a restaurant, a group meeting, or a family gathering, you will be happier with a hearing aid larger than a CIC.

What features do today's hearing aids have to help me hear better?

Hearing aids today come with a wide range of possible features and a wide range of prices. In general, as you go up in price, you're purchasing better technology. This means that you will often get some advanced features in the higher-priced hearing aids that you won't get in lower-priced ones. This is important for you to know because these features will make a big impact on your ability to understand speech in your most challenging listening environments.

The number of possible features can be dizzying. They include automatic volume control, digital noise reduction, directional microphones, features that will make your own voice sound more natural to yourself, features to eliminate squealing sounds, binaural (two-ear) signal processing, frequency-lowering techniques, remote-control features, wireless-streaming options, and water and dust resistance.

Some features, such as automatic volume control, are found in almost every hearing aid on the market. Others, such as binaural signal processing, advanced noise suppression, and the most effective directional microphones will only be found in the most expensive hearing aids. But you may not need to get the most expensive hearing aid on the market—you may be able to economize without giving up performance in your most important listening environments.

To decide whether you need these features, talk with your audiologist about your specific listening requirements and about what you're having difficulty hearing. Your audiologist then can determine which features would most effectively address your individual problems. Also, the audiologist should help determine whether there are features that you do not really need. More features are not always better. Sometimes getting all the different options can be a lot to manage when you just want the hearing aid to adjust to your needs automatically. If you tell your audiologist what you want to accomplish, he or she can select a product that gives you the *results* you need instead of the *features* that sound like a good idea.

What is automatic volume control?

Almost every hearing aid on the market has some sort of automatic volume control. The hearing aid can monitor how loud the incoming sound is and adjust itself based on that. The hearing aid will try to keep soft sounds audible, moderate conversation comfortable, and loud conversation tolerable. When a loud sound comes in, the hearing aid turns the volume down to keep you in your comfort zone. If the room is quiet, the hearing aid pushes the volume a little harder. You never have to touch the volume control; it is automatic. This type of approach will generally keep the hearing aid in your comfort zone 98 percent of the time.

Some people, though, would prefer to control the volume themselves. They prefer a manual volume control, which allows them to make their own decisions about how loud or soft the hearing aid should be in any situation. If you are nervous about having the hearing aid make volume adjustments for you, your audiologist can equip your hearing aid with a small knob or switch to allow you to control the volume yourself. That being said, most people are much more comfortable having the hearing aid make volume adjustments for them.

Many people find the best compromise to be a hybrid device. A hybrid hearing aid has automatic volume control but also gives you the ability to override what the hearing aid thinks you need in situations where you want a little bit more or a little bit less volume.

Is it worth it to get a hearing aid with a directional microphone?

The biggest problem that people have with their hearing loss is hearing while there is background noise. Directional microphones are, by far, the most effective way to deal with that problem. In a noisy environment, directional microphones go into a forward focus. That means they give you your most efficient amplification for what is within eight feet in front of you. In a noisy restaurant, people at your table are generally going to be in front of you and within about eight feet. There also will be a significant amount of noise coming from behind you. In this kind of situation, a hearing aid with a directional microphone will help you focus on the people you want to hear.

It is very important that you understand that no hearing aid can ever simply amplify *only* the things that you want to hear. We don't have a hearing aid that can read your mind. What people typically want to hear with their hearing aids is speech. What they typically want to eliminate also is speech, only this time speech is labeled as background noise because it is a conversation we are not interested in at that moment. A hearing aid in a group of people, though, doesn't know who is interesting and who is boring—or who you would like to hear over the others.

If you're at a party and you want to hear Jim's story, Jim's voice is labeled as speech in your mind. The guy next to him, Joe, is labeled as background noise to you because you don't care about what Joe is saying at that moment. But five minutes later, when you're tired of listening to Jim and want to hear what Joe has to say, now Joe's voice, which used to be background noise, is categorized as speech in your mind. And Jim's voice, which used to be speech, is now labeled background noise. The voices did not change at all. The only thing that changed was who you wanted to listen to. The hearing aid doesn't know when you change your mind about who you are interested in hearing and cannot eliminate the voices just because you consider them boring.

Directional microphones can help solve this problem. With directional microphones, you get your most effective hearing for the person you are facing. In a party environment or a restaurant, you will typically face the person you want to hear, naturally orienting the hearing aid toward the speech you think is most important. So while the hearing aid can't read your mind, it can to an extent read your body language and help you most efficiently amplify the person you are facing.

How does digital noise reduction help?

In the 1990s, the early digital hearing aids tried to amplify only sounds that were behaving like speech and to reduce the amplification for sounds that were not behaving like speech. This feature is called digital noise reduction. Basically, the hearing aids analyzed the number of peaks in volume of the incoming sound. For example, the device would recognize that in running conversation, there are three or four peaks per second in volume. If the incoming sound has a lot more peaks in volume or a lot fewer peaks in volume, the hearing aid would decide that sound is not speech, and it would turn the volume down for those sounds.

Modern hearing devices perform much more sophisticated analyses of the incoming speech sounds than the early devices. They are much more accurate at determining which sounds are acting like speech and which are not. The concept is still the same, though. If a sound behaves like speech, the hearing aid tries to leave the volume turned up; if a sound does not behave like speech, the hearing aid tries to turn the volume down for that particular sound in order to prioritize the important speech signal. Although digital noise reduction helps make noisy situations more tolerable, most of the speech-understanding benefit in the midst of noise comes from the use of directional microphones.

Can I get a feature that will make my own voice sound more natural to myself? Can the annoying sound of my chewing be lessened?

Some of the traditional and common complaints about hearing aids have been "When I'm wearing my hearing aids, my own voice sounds like my head is in a barrel" or "I sound like I'm talking with a bad head cold." Many people say, "My chewing sounds abnormally loud to me when I wear my hearing devices, and it's annoying."

These problems are primarily the result of the hearing aids blocking the ear canals. As you'll recall from our discussion of types of hearing aids, most of this problem can be alleviated with a behind-the-ear hearing aid with its large tunnel or vent. Some hearing aids leave the ear canal so unobstructed that we call them open-fit hearing aids.

What is feedback control, and why might I want it?

Feedback is the squealing that occurs when amplified sound gets re-amplified over and over again. You'll often hear it on public address systems if they're turned up too loud, and a hearing aid is just a miniature public address system.

With hearing aid technology of the past, if we turned up a hearing aid too loud, some of the sound would leak out of the ear canal and get amplified by the hearing aid over and over again. By opening up a large tunnel through the ear canal, as we do with behind-the-ear hearing aids, we open up a path for that sound to leak out of the ear.

Modern hearing devices are able to combat the problem of squealing by incorporating feedback control circuitry that can detect when a hearing aid starts to squeal, at which time it creates an equal but opposite sound, canceling out the squeal. This technology allows us to get more effective power out of the hearing aid without its squealing. A by-product of that is that we are able to open up a large tunnel through the ear canal portion of a behind-the-ear hearing aid without subjecting you to squealing, so that your own voice will sound more natural to you. The development of feedback control technology has essentially made it possible to dramatically increase your ability to hear high-pitched sounds while still making your own voice sound more natural to yourself.

Is a binaural, or two-ear, signal processing feature useful in a hearing aid?

One of the biggest advancements in hearing aid technology in the last few years is the ability of the hearing aids in each of your ears to act as a team to help with noise reduction and increase the clarity of speech in noisy environments. This is called binaural signal process-ing; it essentially means that your two hearing aids communicate with each other dozens of times a second. The right hearing aid talks to the left hearing aid, and the left hearing aid talks to the right hearing aid. If there is a dominant, loud voice on your right side, the hearing aids lower the volume on your left side, allowing you to more effectively focus on the dominant voice.

This feature can be very, very useful if you are trying to listen to one voice in a restaurant or party setting where there is, say, loud chatter on your left side and a dominant voice on your right side. The hearing aids can help coordinate the amplification on the left and the right to help you focus on one ear. This is, in effect, what your ears could do before they had hearing loss. In a noisy environment, your ears could "adjust" their internal volumes, allowing you to focus on one side or the other. Modern hearing aids with binaural signal processing can approximate that effect, although not as well as your natural biology could before you had hearing loss.

Could I be helped by frequency-lowering techniques?

In some kinds of hearing losses, people have frequencies or pitches at which the hearing loss is so severe that no matter how loud we make sounds, they will not be clear. Essentially, there's a blind spot in the hearing. This effect typically occurs at high pitches and often is caused by years of exposure to loud noise. In people with blind spots in their hearing, no matter how loud a hearing device makes high-pitched sounds, such as *s, f,* and *th*, the ear and brain will not hear them.

For people with blind spots in their hearing, hearing aid technology can take those high pitches and shift them to lower pitches at which the person's hearing is better. Patients often say that, initially, the lowered speech sounds are a little distorted, lispy, or slushy but that usually after four to six weeks, those sounds start to become more natural. The brain starts to accommodate the sounds and use them to be able to understand speech more effectively than it could with traditional amplification.

Do you recommend remote controls for hearing aids?

Some hearing aids have various settings the user can control. For example, you may prefer to get a hearing aid that allows you to switch on a music-appreciation mode or a background-noise-reduction mode yourself rather than have your hearing aid do it automatically. Some users like to be able to manually control the volume of their hearing aids by pressing + or –. Most hearing devices are available with all of the controls on board the hearing aid itself, the controls in a remote-control device, or both.

If you have a hearing aid that allows you to change settings, remote controls give you easy access to those different settings in your hearing aid. I have to admit that I have a love-hate relationship with remote controls for hearing aids. They can be incredibly useful for some patients and just an expensive gimmick for others.

Before you get a hearing aid that you adjust using a remote device, think about this: having all of the controls and adjustments available on the hearing aids themselves is incredibly convenient. If you're wearing the hearing aid, you have full access to all of its features at any time. You don't have to remember to bring your remote control with you when you go out or even go to another room in your house; you still have the ability to change the volume or to make adjustments to your hearing aids.

If you do not have good manual dexterity—for example, if you have arthritis or numbness in your fingers—or have vision problems, a remote-control device can be a very useful option. A remote control is easier to manipulate. You do have to carry it with you, but if you physically cannot make the adjustments you'd like on your hearing aids, a remote can be very helpful.

My experience has been that most patients absolutely love the remote control for three weeks. Then they get tired of carrying it around with them, and it ends up sitting on the nightstand at home. This means the hearing aid wearer does not have the ability to adjust the hearing aids except in bed—which is not very useful.

If you're getting a hearing aid with a remote control, then I'd advise you to make sure the hearing aid also has onboard adjustments as well. That way, if you forget your remote at home or decide not to carry it with you, you still have the ability to control the hearing aid by using the buttons or controls mounted directly on it.

Why might wireless streaming options be useful?

Modern hearing aids can now be set up to act as wireless headphones for a number of different sound sources. You might have sound sent directly from your cell phone, TV, computer, iPad, MP3 player, or stereo to your hearing aids, in essence turning them into a set of earphones that make the sound much clearer. This is similar to using a Bluetooth earpiece with your cell phone. The difference is that the audio signal can be sent to both ears and amplified by the hearing aid to dramatically improve the clarity.

Almost every major hearing aid manufacturer currently has the option of a wireless streaming device for use with your hearing aids. The wonderful thing is that you, the hearing aid wearer, can then have individual control over how loud you want to hear an electronic sound source. If you're watching television with your spouse and want to turn up the volume, you can do so using the wireless streaming option for your hearing aid, and your spouse can listen at the volume desired. This option, obviously, can eliminate a lot of arguments in the home over the desired TV volume.

Would any features be able to help with my tinnitus?

Many people with and without hearing loss are bothered by tinnitus, a sound that you can hear but that is not actually in the world around you. Buzzing, roaring, ringing, hissing, or thumping noises are commonly reported.

As we said in chapter 6, if you have tinnitus and also need hearing aids, just wearing the hearing aids may be enough to interrupt tinnitus and provide relief, but tinnitus instruments (devices that combine hearing aid and tinnitus sound therapy) might be helpful. These devices act as hearing aids but also can be programmed to deliver an interfering noise through the earpiece—usually static or a semi-musical sound—to cover up the tinnitus or distract you from it when you want it to. Your brain is able to stop focusing on the tinnitus and stop viewing it as a threat or a danger, which in turn allows you to push the tinnitus into your subconscious.

Should I look for a hearing aid with water and dust resistance?

Today's hearing aids are much more resistant to water, dirt, and dust than in the past. Most hearing aids now are designed to be water-resistant, which means they can tolerate a brief submersion in one meter of water. In practical terms, that means if you got your hearing aid wet or even dunked it under water as deep as three feet, it would probably come back to life if you opened up the battery compartment and let it dry out for a day or two.

You might be wondering why depth of water is more important than how long a hearing aid is underwater. The deeper the water, the more force the water pressure exerts on the hearing aid, and the more likely it is that water will infiltrate the hearing aid.

Since most hearing aids are water-resistant, they will stand up to brief exposure to water or rain. For example, if you get caught in the rain or forget to remove them before showering, they should be fine as long as you open them up, take out the battery, and let them dry out. Still, even though they are designed to withstand brief exposures to water, try not to put your hearing aids to the test.

Some people would like even more water-resistance. If you participate in activities that run the risk of getting submerged in water—fishing, white-water rafting, kayaking—you may want to order waterproof hearing aids. These hearing aids continue to run even after submersion in water and are rated to even greater depths of submersion. Some are rated as submersible in three to nine meters of water and will still function when you take them out to dry.

If you choose waterproof hearing aids, however, be aware that you probably will have to make some sacrifices in sound quality. You may have to trade off some of the sound-processing strategies we normally use for improved clarity in order to get a waterproof hearing aid.

What Can I Expect from My Hearing Aids?

- cosmetics you feel good about
- improved speech understanding, even in moderately noisy environments like the car and in restaurants

- easier communication at a distance, including across the room, in a classroom, or in a lecture setting
- little to no whistling, squealing, or feedback
- comfort that allows you to wear them most waking hours of the day without thinking much about them
- audible soft speech, comfortable conversational speech, tolerable loud speech
- improved quality of life

How can I choose one brand or manufacturer over all the others?

At this time, approximately seven manufacturers make the vast majority of hearing aids sold in the United States. The truth is, every single one of these manufacturers makes a good-quality product. But they differ in their ideas about what someone with a hearing loss needs in terms of sound processing.

The truth is that no one manufacturer makes the right hearing aid for everyone, but each one makes the right hearing aid for someone. Therefore, when choosing a hearing aid, be sure that you go to an audiologist who carries several manufacturers' brands. These audiologists will be able to advise you—based on your hearing test—which manufacturer is most likely to fit your needs; they will try to find the right hearing aid for you rather than trying to fit your hearing loss into what one manufacturer has to offer. Chapter 2 gave other tips on finding a great audiologist for your needs.

CHAPTER 8

What Insurance Coverage and Legal Protections Will I Have When I Purchase Hearing Aids?

I n spite of my office's best efforts to make sure that everyone understands their protections in buying hearing aids, almost every year a situation comes up that could have been avoided. Recently, a patient, who I'll call Sarah, came in and told me that she had purchased hearing aids about five years earlier. Sadly, about three months into wearing the hearing aids, her dog ate them—crushed them beyond recognition. She was devastated. The hearing aids had been a huge help. They had improved the quality of her life dramatically. But they were expensive. She knew she couldn't afford a second pair and just suffered in silence as she saved her money for the next set. Now, five years later, Sarah finally had enough money and came in to see me to get her next set of hearing devices.

If she had only known that almost every hearing device sold in the United States comes with loss and damage insurance! This means that in that first year of ownership, she could have gone back to her hearing aid provider and got a brand new replacement set of hearing aids for little or no cost.

Every hearing aid sold in the United States will come with a printed list of all of your rights—your right to free repairs, your right to replacement in the event of loss or a dog eating the hearing aids, and your right to return the hearing aids for a refund. Be sure you read this information when you get your hearing aids. You will be presented with an enormous amount of information when you first get your hearing device, but your rights are among the most important part of this information.

This chapter outlines your rights when you buy a hearing device. A number of legal protections ensure that your hearing aids are successful for you and that you are successful with them. The bottom line is that if there's ever a problem with your hearing devices—even if you lose them, you run them over with a car, or the dog eats them—get in touch with your audiologist and find out what protection you have.

Hearing aids are a major expense. Your insurance provider may cover a portion of the purchase price. In addition, the hearing aid industry is regulated by the government, and a number of laws exist to protect you, the consumer, as you purchase your hearing aids. Understanding your legal protections will help you get the hearing aids that are best for you.

How can I know if my insurance will cover anything related to my hearing aids?

Almost 30 percent of the new patients in my office have some form of hearing aid coverage through their health insurance. The insurance usually doesn't cover the entire cost of hearing aids, but it often covers $1,000 to $4,000, which is certainly a big chunk of the hearing aid purchase.

When you call in to consider an appointment with an audiologist's office, be sure to tell them what health insurance you have. You will want to find out if that office is what's called a preferred provider for your insurance. If they are a preferred provider, it means that they are contracted with your insurance company to give you the best possible price to maximize your insurance benefits. This may mean that the co-pays are lower or that your deductible is lower. In some cases, in fact, your insurance may *only* provide a benefit if you go to a preferred provider. You may find out that your insurance company will not pay for you to go to the first office you call. Therefore, it is important to discuss your insurance before you make an appointment to go in for a hearing test.

Be sure to ask the audiologist's office up front whether your insurance will cover the cost of your exam, and ask them to find out if the hearing devices would be covered as well. That way, when you're figuring out what device you want to purchase, you will have a clear understanding of what your out-of-pocket costs will be.

I have Medicare. What will it cover in relation to my hearing aids?

Medicare typically covers the cost of a hearing test if it is medically necessary. It will not cover the cost of hearing aids, however. It also does not cover routine exams (exams that are not medically necessary). And, unfortunately, the definition of *medically necessary* is not clear-cut.

In general, though, if you tell your primary care doctor that you are truly concerned about your hearing and you would like a hearing test to find out whether medical treatment is available, you should get a referral for a hearing test that Medicare will cover.

Medicare will not cover hearing tests solely for the purpose of getting a hearing aid. This means that if you know that you have a hearing loss already, and you know that it is not medically treatable, but instead you want a hearing aid, Medicare will probably not cover your hearing exam. However, if you suspect you have a hearing loss and want to find out what all your treatment options are, Medicare typically will cover the cost of the exam.

The preceding discussion assumes that Medicare is your primary insurance. If you have a Medicare Replacement Plan (often called a MedAdvantage plan) instead of Medicare—for example, Blue Cross Blue Shield's Medicare Advantage or Providence Health's Medicare Replacement Plan—you might have a hearing aid benefit or partial coverage for a hearing aid purchase.

What to ask your insurance carrier before you get hearing aids or, better yet, before you sign up or renew your plan:

1. Is hearing health care covered under this plan? (If not, ask if they have a similar one that is covered.)

2. Are there any age restrictions on who can exercise this hearing aid benefit? (It will do you no good if they only cover hearing aids for children and you're forty-five.)

3. What kind of deductible will I need to meet in order to have you pay out on a hearing aid claim?

4. What is the allowable maximum for hearing care under this plan?

5. What kind of co-pay will I be expected to pay?

6. Can I see any provider or does it have to be one in your network?

7. Does this plan cover repairs, batteries, or replacement?

What if I decide not to get hearing aids after I take a hearing test? What will I have to pay?

Any reputable audiologist will charge for a hearing test. The office should be willing to tell you the cost for the exam prior to your appointment.

Hearing testing is not terribly expensive. It's probably the cheapest part of the process of getting hearing devices. Do not decide whether to go to a particular provider based on how much the initial hearing test will cost. Newspaper ads may tout free hearing tests, but ask yourself, "How is this person making a living?" No one can make a living giving free hearing tests 100 percent of their time. *If you are considering going to providers who are advertising a free hearing test, keep in mind that the only way that they can make their paycheck that month is if they convince you to buy a hearing aid, whether you need it or not.*

When you go to an audiologist to talk about hearing aids, you should be prepared to actually pay for that time with the provider. In the end, being willing to pay a small amount for a hearing test will better ensure that you will get honest, unbiased opinions about whether it's time to get a hearing aid.

What if I don't like my hearing aids after I get them?

Patients sometimes come into my office with the same complaint: "I bought a set of hearing aids, but they don't work for me, so I just put them in the drawer."

This should never happen. You should never, ever be one of these patients who buys a hearing aid and winds up putting it in a drawer because you do not like it. A number of laws protect you, the consumer, when you buy hearing aids. This following section on legal protections discusses some of the most important protections that you have in buying hearing aids so that they stay in your ear and not in the drawer.

What legal protections do I have when I purchase hearing aids?

The US hearing aid industry is regulated by a number of laws. When you purchase new hearing aids, you must receive a trial period and will almost certainly receive a warranty period and a loss and damage insurance period. Read on to learn about your legal rights in each of these periods. If you are aware of your rights, you will be protected from purchasing hearing aids that do not work for you.

How does the trial period for my hearing aids protect me?

Every hearing aid sold in the United States comes with a trial period. This is a period of time during which you can try out the hearing aid in your real-world situation—in your daily life—and decide whether this hearing aid is making your quality of life better. You can learn how your hearing aid sounds at home, at work, and anywhere else you go. In short, you have this time to decide whether or not you would like to keep the hearing device or return it for a refund.

Federal law specifies that you must have a minimum of thirty days to try out your hearing aid. It's not uncommon to find a sixty-day trial period, and occasionally you'll find an office that will give a ninety-day trial period. During that period of time, if you decide that you don't want to keep the hearing aid for any reason, you may return it for a refund.

If you do return the hearing aid for a refund during your trial period, you should expect a few expenses that may not be refundable. Typically, the cost of the hearing test is not refundable, although in some states if you return a hearing aid the hearing test charge may also be refunded.

Most states allow the audiologist to retain a small amount of the purchase price as a restocking fee to cover things like the audiologist's time and shipping costs. This is always specified in state law. Most states put a cap on the amount of money that the audiologist can hold back in the event of a hearing aid return. Some states cap the restocking fee by a dollar amount, such as one hundred dollars per hearing aid; other states will specify the restocking fee in a percentage, as in up to 10 percent of the purchase price of the hearing aid.

Your purchase agreement should specify any restocking fee or other nonrefundable fees. Your audiologist will give you these details for that specific office.

What does my hearing aid's warranty mean to me?

Hearing aids typically come with a one-, two-, or three-year warranty. During this time, the manufacturer must fix any problems with the hearing aid. These repairs should cover things like earwax working its way into the hearing aid or accidental moisture damage. It should cover repairs if your hearing aid just doesn't sound right, the hearing aid works intermittently or sounds distorted, or the device stops working for any reason. These types of repairs are considered normal wear and tear, and your warranty should cover them in full during that first one to three years.

You can purchase extended warranties for hearing aids. Most manufacturers will extend the hearing aid warranty out to as long as five years. You can expect to spend a few hundred dollars per year to extend the warranty on a pair of high-tech hearing aids.

I am not a big fan of extended warranties, because hearing aids are fairly durable. If you take reasonable care of them, you'll generally spend less on hearing aid repairs throughout the lifetime of the device than you would on extended warranties. If I were in your shoes, I would simply put a couple of hundred dollars a year into a savings account and pay for your repairs out of that money. At the end of the lifespan of your hearing aid, say five years, you'll usually be several hundred dollars ahead.

How does the loss and damage insurance period for my hearing aids help me?

Your hearing aids, by law, come with a loss and damage insurance period. This is separate from your hearing aid warranty and is designed to cover severe abuse and neglect. Loss and damage insurance is designed to provide you with some protection if you lose the hearing aid or it sustains catastrophic damage. You will be covered if your hearing aid is lost, burned up in a fire, or fed to the dog. You could eat it, beat it to death with a sledgehammer, or drop it down the garbage disposal. You would be surprised at what people do to their hearing aids.

So even if you have obviously abused or neglected your hearing aid, and even if the hearing aid comes back to the audiologist in fifteen pieces, your loss and damage insurance will provide a new hearing aid during the loss and damage period. This period is typically one to two years, and this kind of insurance typically comes standard in a new hearing aid purchase. The loss and damage insurance typically covers one replacement on each hearing aid during the insurance period. If you lose your right hearing aid and have it replaced, you still have coverage on your left hearing aid during this period.

Most loss and damage insurance policies have a deductible to pay the claim. It may be a dollar amount, such as $150 per hearing aid, or it may be a percentage, such as 10 percent of the purchase price of the hearing aid. But certainly, in the event of a catastrophic event, a deductible is much, much less expensive than buying a whole new hearing aid.

The bottom line is that if you lose or crush your hearing aid, don't panic. Call your audiologist. Find out if you still have loss and damage insurance, and see if you're eligible for a replacement. There's a limited time to do this, and the clock is ticking, so don't delay. Nothing is worse than having somebody come into my office and tell me they lost their new hearing aid two years ago and that now they're ready to buy a new one. They simply could have had a replacement provided at little to no cost had they acted right away.

Loss and damage insurance can be extended beyond the first few years through the original hearing aid manufacturer or a third-party insurance company. Again, I'm not a huge fan of buying extended loss and damage policies. Extended loss and damage insurance tends to be fairly expensive. If you're a reasonably responsible adult, you will probably keep good track of your hearing aids, especially if you're a full-time hearing aid user. However, if you are worried about losing or damaging your hearing aids and the expense involved with replacing them, you might want to consider purchasing extended loss and damage insurance. For example, if you're blind, if the hearing aids belong to a child, if you're in assisted living, or if you have memory problems or tend to lose your glasses and keys, extended loss and damage insurance may be perfect for you.

An alternative to loss and damage insurance that many people don't think about is itemizing your hearing aids on your homeowners or renters insurance policy. Homeowners insurance or renters insurance tends to have a much cheaper yearly premium to insure your hearing aids, but you will probably face a much higher deductible in the event of a loss.

Do I have any protection if my hearing aids suddenly stop working well after the trial or warranty period?

It is common for hearing aids to suddenly stop working well at some point in their lifespan. They may have been perfectly satisfactory for two or three years, but then you notice that the device sounds weak, dead, or just odd. This situation can be due to a few different things.

Your hearing may have changed. After all, hearing changes all the time. Hearing loss typically is a slowly progressing condition, but it does tend to get worse over time. If you have a pair of hearing aids that seem to be gradually getting worse and worse, your hearing loss may have outgrown the current settings in the hearing aids.

You should be getting your hearing tested every one to two years, at a minimum. If your hearing loss has worsened, usually your hearing aid can be reprogrammed or readjusted to match those changes in your hearing loss. Talk with your audiologist and set up an appropriate hearing testing schedule. If you visit your audiologist only when there's a problem, you can easily lose five or six years of improved quality of life by not addressing the changes in your hearing loss.

The other common reason hearing aids stop working well is due to mechanical problems. Most of these problems can be addressed very, very quickly. The most common problem that occurs suddenly is earwax getting embedded into the part of the hearing aid that allows sound to reach your eardrum. This problem is usually very, very easy to fix. If you have a hearing aid that was sounding great yesterday and today it sounds dead, your audiologist usually will be able to bring the hearing aid back to life in five minutes or less.

Sometimes a hearing aid has become so impacted with earwax that it has to be sent to the manufacturer for some new components. Even that, however, is a relatively easy procedure and much cheaper than getting a brand new hearing aid.

In general, if your hearing aid is five years old or less, you can expect it to be easily repairable and easily adjustable for your hearing-loss changes. Never sit at home frustrated. If you have a problem, pick up the phone and call your audiologist. You're not being a nuisance. You are simply letting your audiologist know that you need some help. Your job as a hearing aid wearer is to be proactive. If you have a problem with your hearing aid, talk about it with your provider. It probably will help—and it certainly can't hurt.

CONCLUSION

What Am I Waiting For?

With all of the benefits to diagnosing and treating your hearing loss early, I hope you agree that it's never been a better time for you to start doing something about it. By reading his book, you have already come one big step closer to improving your life.

I can't stress it enough—if you have hearing loss, using hearing aids can dramatically improve almost every quality-of-life measure: mental health, physical health, earning potential, relationships, and work performance. And with satisfaction rates over 85 percent, why wait to increase your confidence and independence? Whether you've just turned twenty-seven or eighty-seven, you owe it to yourself to determine what may be holding you back and start moving forward.

You now have the knowledge to start getting back in the driver's seat. You know the basics about hearing loss and hearing aids, and you are armed with the right questions to ask and feel confident enough to ask them. You now know what to look for in a qualified audiologist, so you will be an integral part of the process when it is time to get your hearing tested. Hearing aids are a life-changing event, and by reading this book, you can now get those benefits for yourself.

It is time to pick up the phone and call your audiologist, get a hearing test, and listen to what hearing devices can do for you. There's no reason to be yet another person who puts this off for years and years as your brain becomes less and less able to handle sound. Remember, you are in control of your health care.

If you have any questions, wish to discuss anything you have read in this book in more detail, or would like to contact me for a hearing consultation area, please use the information below to contact me. If you are outside of the Portland, Oregon, area, I strongly encourage you to contact a local audiologist for a hearing test and hearing consultation. The next step is to pick up the phone and call, and that step is up to you.

Eric Frederick, AuD
Audiology Center Northwest
(503) 232-1845
customerservice@audiologycenternw.com
www.audiologycenternw.com

GLOSSARY

air conduction. The presentation of sound by moving air molecules. This is accomplished with earphones or loudspeakers. We normally hear through air conduction. This type of testing requires sound to travel through all three parts of your ear, the outer, middle, and inner ear, before you can hear it. Any problems in any of these three areas will affect your air-conduction hearing.

amplification. In our context, it is the act of making something louder. Amplification is sometimes used as another word for a hearing aid.

assistive listening device (ALD). Any non-hearing aid device designed to help you hear or detect a sound. This could include a battery-powered personal amplifier, a telephone amplifier, a flashing light to alert you to a doorbell or fire alarm, a vibrator to shake your pillow to wake you up if you cannot hear the alarm clock, etc.

audiogram. A graph which indicates the softest sound you can hear for several different pitches. The audiogram is typically performed without hearing aids being worn to determine whether you have a hearing loss. Specific patterns of results on the audiogram can also help your audiologist understand what part of your ear may be affected by your hearing loss.

audiologist. A university-trained professional with specific expertise in hearing, hearing loss, hearing aids, and vestibular and balance testing. Any new audiologist in the United States must now have a doctorate degree to begin practice. That is usually a doctor of audiology (AuD) degree, but you may occasionally see an audiologist with a PhD or ScD degree as well. In the past, audiologists were able to practice with only a master's degree. You may see some audiologists still practicing with an MA or MS degree. That simply means they have been practicing since before the more stringent requirements for a doctoral degree were enacted for audiologists.

bone-anchored hearing aid. A hearing device that is installed by a surgeon. It is usually used to treat either a conductive hearing loss or hearing loss where one ear is essentially deaf, but the other is near normal. This device is not typically appropriate for the most common type of hearing loss, sensorineural hearing loss on both sides.

bone conduction. Testing that is performed by vibrating the bones of the skull instead of vibrating air molecules. Instead of testing with earphones or loudspeakers, a small vibrator box is placed behind the ear or on the forehead. The vibrations travel through the skull to the inner ear. This allows the audiologist to determine whether the hearing loss is due to a problem in the inner ear versus a problem in the middle/outer ear area. This information is vital to determine whether surgery may be a viable treatment.

BTE. Behind-the-ear hearing aid. This type of hearing aid has all of the electronic components of the hearing aid worn over the top of the ear with a small wire or tube leading to an earmold or earplug that sits in the ear canal.

CIC. Completely-in-the-canal hearing aid. This type of hearing aid has all of the electronic components of the hearing aid worn inside of the ear canal. This style of hearing aid fills the entire ear canal but does not extend into the outer portion of the ear. This style of hearing aid is cosmetically appealing but may not be able to provide as much power for severe hearing losses as an ITE or BTE style.

cochlea. The inner ear. This is the portion of the ear that converts sound from mechanical movement into an electrical signal that can be sent up to the auditory nerve to the brain. This is the part of the hearing system that is most often damaged with sensorineural hearing loss. In addition, your vestibular function, which is vital to your ability to balance and stay upright, is located in the cochlea.

cochlear implant. A surgically implanted hearing device used for very severe hearing loss. This device stimulates the auditory nerve with electricity instead of sound. This device is generally used when the hearing loss is so severe that hearing aids cannot provide benefit.

conductive hearing loss. A hearing loss located in the outer or middle ears. This type of hearing loss occurs when the mechanical vibration of sound is damped down. In this type of hearing loss, the inner ear, or cochlea is still functioning well.

decibel (dB). A measure of sound intensity. For most people, higher numbers mean louder sounds. For instance, a whisper may only be 20–30 decibels, but a gunshot may be 130–140 decibels.

ear, nose, and throat physician (ENT). Some other names you may see for this highly trained professional are otolaryngologist (ear, nose, throat), otologist (ears only), or neurotologist (ears and brain). All of these refer to medical doctors who are trained to treat hearing loss. Their training specifically includes medications and surgeries but carries only a little training on hearing aids themselves.

hearing aid. A device worn on or in the ear that is specifically programmed or tuned for your individual hearing loss. This is not a "one-size-fits-all" device but is fitted by prescription to meet your individual needs. This type of device is designed for hearing-impaired people with the intention of treating their hearing loss.

hearing aid dealer. Sometimes referred to as a hearing instrument specialist, hearing instrument dealer, or occasionally an audioprothetologist. In most states, these are retail sales people. Some states require some university-level training; others do not. In general, the most rigorous training of hearing aid dealers result in BC-HIS after their name. Even with that designation, an audiologist will usually have six additional years of university training beyond the BC-HIS requirements.

IIC. An even smaller version of the completely-in-the-canal hearing aid that fits even deeper than the CIC style. This type of hearing aid has all of the electronic components of the hearing aid worn inside of the ear canal. This style of hearing aid fills the entire ear canal but does not extend into the outer portion of the ear. This style of hearing aid is cosmetically appealing but may not be able to provide as much power for severe hearing losses as an ITE or BTE style. In addition, many ear canals may not be large enough or shaped in a way that will allow an IIC fitting.

ITC. In-the-ear hearing aid. This type of hearing aid has all of the electronic components of the hearing aid worn inside of the ear. This style of hearing aid fills the lower one third of the bowl-shaped portion of the ear and is significantly smaller than the ITE style but may not be able to provide as much power for severe hearing losses as an ITE or BTE style.

ITE. In-the-ear hearing aid. This type of hearing aid has all of the electronic components of the hearing aid worn inside of the ear. This style of hearing aid fills the entire bowl-shaped portion of the ear and is generally the most noticeable of all the styles when worn.

lip-reading. The act of trying to understand speech by watching the shape of the lips and mouth. Lip-reading is a very difficult task and one that generally provides very poor levels of understanding.

loss and damage insurance. An insurance policy issued with almost all new hearing aids. The insurance may be used to get a replacement hearing aid in the event that a hearing aid was damaged beyond repair due to severe abuse or neglect. Some examples of events that would be covered by this insurance are losing the hearing aid, the dog ate the hearing aid, the hearing aid was crushed, etc. Most loss and damage insurances require a small fee to get a replacement hearing aid.

mBTE. Mini behind-the-ear hearing aid. This smaller version of the BTE hearing aid has all of the electronic components of the hearing aid worn over the top of the ear with a small wire or tube leading to an earmold or earplug that sits in the ear canal.

mRITE. Mini receiver-in-the-ear hearing aid. This is a specific, smaller type of the BTE or RITE style of hearing aid that has most of the electronic components of the hearing aid worn over the top of the ear with a small wire or leading to an earmold or earplug that sits in the ear canal. The thing that makes the RITE or mRITE styles of hearing aid different from the BTE styles is that the loudspeaker, sometimes called the receiver, sits inside the ear canal instead of on top of the ear.

otolaryngologist. Ear, nose and throat physician.

provider. A generic term that refers to any professional that is providing hearing testing or hearing aids. This could include audiologists, hearing aid dealers, or ENTs.

pure tone. This is a very specific type of sound that is designed to emit just one frequency or pitch. We use this to stimulate a very specific part of the ear. Pure tones generally sound like beeps to the listener.

RIC. Receiver-in-the-canal hearing aid. RIC is an interchangeable synonym with RITE. This is a specific type of the BTE or RITE style of hearing aid that has most of the electronic components of the hearing aid worn over the top of the ear with a small wire or leading to an earmold or earplug that sits in the ear canal. The thing that makes the RIC style of hearing aid different from the BTE styles is that the loudspeaker, sometimes called the receiver, sits inside the ear canal instead of on top of the ear.

RITE. Receiver-in-the-ear hearing aid. This is a specific type of the BTE or RITE style of hearing aid that has most of the electronic components of the hearing aid worn over the top of the ear with a small wire or leading to an earmold or earplug that sits in the ear canal. The thing that makes the RITE or mRITE styles of hearing aid different from the BTE styles is that the loudspeaker, sometimes called the receiver, sits inside the ear canal instead of on top of the ear.

sensorineural hearing loss. Hearing loss located in the inner ear, auditory nerve, or brain. This type of hearing loss is almost always permanent and is typically treated with hearing aids or cochlear implants. The most common type of sensorineural hearing loss is a loss of cells in the cochlea.

speechreading. Often confused with lipreading. This is the act of watching a combination of a person's lips, gestures, and facial expressions. This information can be used to enhance whatever portion of speech the person is able to hear.

trial period. The period of time after purchase during which you may return the hearing aid for a refund. Federal regulations require a minimum of thirty-day trial period in the US. There may be a restocking fee associated with returning a hearing aid during this period.

warranty. The policy that covers repairs on the hearing aid resulting from normal wear and use of the hearing aid.

CPSIA information can be obtained at www.ICGtesting.com
Printed in the USA
BVOW06s0109030816

R7249900001B/R72499PG457457BVX6B/8/P